OXFORD MEDICAL PUBLICATONS

Contraception

THE FACTS

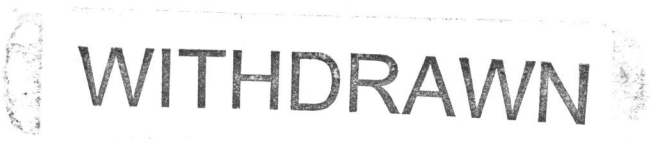

Contraception

THE FACTS

PETER BROMWICH
Clinical Lecturer,
Nuffield Department of Obstetrics and Gynaecology,
John Radcliffe Hospital, University of Oxford

and

TONY PARSONS
Lecturer in Gynaecology,
Department of Obstetrics and Gynaecology,
University of Birmingham

OXFORD NEW YORK TORONTO
OXFORD UNIVERSITY PRESS
1984

Oxford University Press, Walton Street, Oxford OX2 6DP
London New York Toronto
Delhi Bombay Calcutta Madras Karachi
Kuala Lumpur Singapore Hong Kong Tokyo
Nairobi Dar es Salaam Cape Town
Melbourne Auckland
and associated companies in
Beirut Berlin Ibadan Mexico City Nicosia

Oxford is a trade mark of Oxford University Press

British Library Cataloguing in Publication Data
Bromwich, Peter
Contraception.—(Oxford medical publications)
1. Contraception
I. Title II. Parsons, Tony
613.9'4 RG136
ISBN 0-19-261410-X

Library of Congress Cataloguing in Publication Data
Bromwich, Peter.
Contraception: the facts.
(Oxford medical publications)
Includes index.
1. Contraception. I. Parsons, Tony (Antony David)
II. Title. III. Series.
RG136.B696 1984 613.9'4 84-5698
ISBN 0-19-261410-X

Printed in Great Britain by
Richard Clay (The Chaucer Press) Ltd
Bungay, Suffolk

Contents

1

Introduction

This book is about contraception. It deals with all the available methods of preventing or stopping an unwanted pregnancy. It also describes how these methods might fail, how you might find yourself pregnant, and what to do if this happens. But before we discuss ways of stopping pregnancies, we will first give a brief description of reproductive anatomy and the cycle leading to pregnancy. Some readers may wish to skip this summary and go straight on to the discussion of contraception which begins on p.7

Reproduction in women
The ovaries

Women produce an egg on average once a month. These eggs develop from the ovaries, of which there are two, one on each side of the lower abdomen. Each ovary contains the potential for many millions of eggs. These potential eggs are formed in the first few weeks of the woman's life after her conception. From then on the process is one of wastage; only about 400 eggs are released during the whole of her life and most of the potential eggs have disappeared by the time she is born.

Egg development is under the control of the pituitary gland, which itself is controlled by the hypothalamus, which is that part of the brain immediately adjacent to it. Small pulses of hormones from the pituitary act on the ovary and choose a small group of eggs to begin developing. One of these eggs becomes dominant, and its growth outstrips that of all the others. It forms a hormone-secreting layer of cells around it (the follicle), and these hormones act on almost every other cell of the body, directly or indirectly. From the

Contraception: the facts

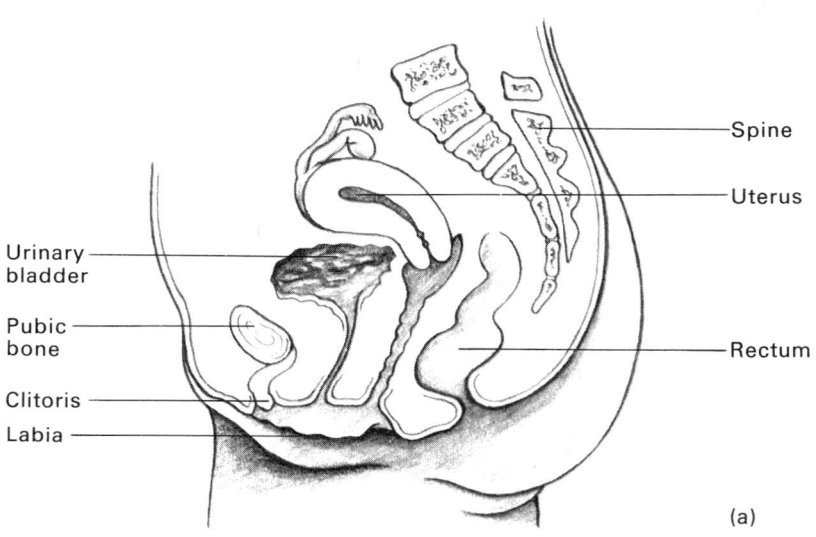

Spine
Uterus
Urinary bladder
Pubic bone
Clitoris
Labia
Rectum

(a)

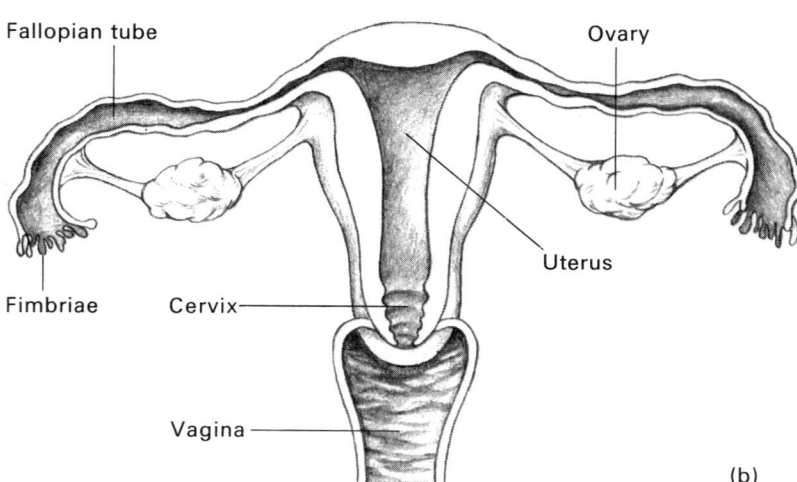

Fallopian tube
Ovary
Fimbriae
Cervix
Uterus
Vagina

(b)

Fig. 1.

Introduction

point of view of reproduction the most important actions are on the cervix and the endometrium.

About 16 days before the next period is due (that is about two days before the egg is due to be released) the rising levels of oestrogen from the developing follicle trigger off a surge of hormone from the pituitary. This surge of *L*uteinizing *H*ormone (more usually known as LH) is enough to change the quality of the tissue covering the follicle, making it thinner so that the follicle bursts at this weakened spot, releasing the egg and the cells that surround it into the Fallopian tube. The cycle has begun.

The Fallopian tubes

There are two of these, one leading from each of the two ovaries into each side of the womb. They are hollow, and the ends that cover the ovaries have very finely formed hairs, or fronds (the fimbriae) which help to waft the mature egg from the surface of the ovary into the tube. If the fimbriae are damaged by disease or surgery they are unable to collect the egg, and the meeting of the egg and sperm becomes much less likely. Many scientists think that the fluid secreted by the tubal lining is essential for normal functioning of the sperms and the eggs, and if this lining is damaged by infection this might be the explanation for some cases of infertility.

If the mature egg is successfully wafted along the tube, and intercourse has taken place within the last few days, it may meet and fuse with a sperm that has worked its way along to the Fallopian tube. This fusion is called fertilization. The fertilized egg will then be wafted along the rest of the tube and into the womb where it will begin to bury itself in the lining and start to develop. However, most fertilizations do not develop any further and the woman will not be aware that anything out of the ordinary is happening—the egg will be passed out with the lining of the womb during the next menstrual period.

3

The cervix

The sperms reach the Fallopian tubes by passing up the vagina and through the neck of the womb—the cervix. This smooth, firm structure forms a barrier between the organs buried inside the body and those that are open to the outside. It has an extremely important role in keeping the internal organs free from infection, and yet at the same time allows enough sperms into the Fallopian tubes to let fertilization happen. It keeps the womb closed during pregnancy, but gradually stretches during labour to allow the baby to be born.

These different functions mean that the anatomy of the cervix has to be complex and yet capable of rapid change. It has a firm fibrous base to give it strength, but the fibres soften and stretch by taking in water under the influence of hormones. This softening and swelling is most noticeable during pregnancy, but can sometimes be detected during the normal hormonal changes that accompany ovulation. The outer lining of the cervix has a layer of cells that secrete mucus, which changes in nature throughout the menstrual cycle. The surface is heaped into many—perhaps one hundred—small hills and valleys, and the fibres of mucus from each individual pocket or crypt tend to align. This produces long strands of mucus, and spermatozoa swim up the strands away from the vagina, which is too acid for them to live in. This ideal mucus is produced in response to hormones secreted by the egg and its follicle as they develop in the ovary. It is at its peak for only one to four days in each month, shortly before the time that an egg is released, and more than twenty times as much of it is produced than on other days. This mucus is essential for normal survival and development of sperms. During the rest of the cycle little mucus is produced, and what there is tends to consist of densely interwoven and impenetrable strands which keep spermatozoa away from the internal organs. It has none of the nutrient factors that sperm need to survive and mature,

4

and so by looking at your mucus and timing intercourse you can make a pregnancy less likely to occur.

Reproduction in men

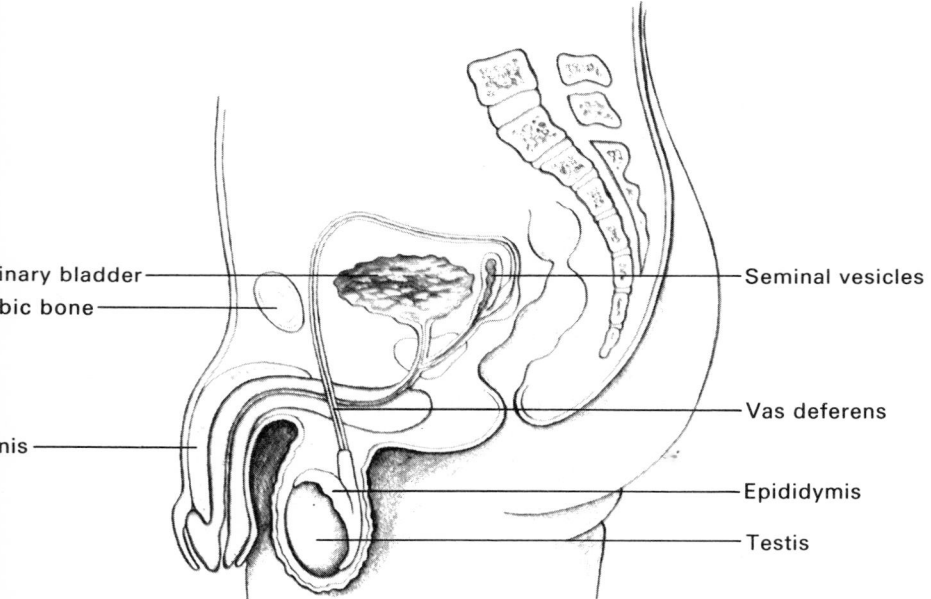

inary bladder

bic bone

nis

Seminal vesicles

Vas deferens

Epididymis

Testis

Fig. 2

The testes or testicles

There are two testes that are suspended in a skin-covered bag, the scrotum. Unlike women, who are born with all of the eggs they are ever going to release, men start producing sperms at puberty, and carry on producing new ones for the rest of their lives. The testes consist of three-quarters of a mile of tightly packed tubes, and the sperms are produced in a continuous process on the inner lining of the tubes. When they have been formed they drop into the tube, and pass along to the epididymis.

The epididymis

This is a small tubular structure on the upper edge of the testis. Sperms live in here for about twelve days, and undergo their final maturing process. It is here that they gain the ability to fertilize eggs, and the ability to swim. There are many delicate biological processes that occur here, and it may be possible in years to come to find a way of blocking these changes, and so have a male contraceptive.

The vas deferens

Each epididymis leads into a long tube that leads past the seminal vesicles and through the prostate gland. Both of these glands provide some of the secretions that make up the male ejaculatory fluid, and might also provide some of the nutrient factors that help sperm to function normally. The tubes are long, and for part of their journey to the outside are very close to the skin. This makes it easy to block them surgically in the procedure known as vasectomy. The two tubes join together with the outlet tube from the bladder to form one duct, that runs along the length of the penis to the outside.

The penis

The penis has two functions. It is used for urination, and for sex. It has the ability to grow and become rigid when men are sexually aroused, and it is this property that allows sperms to be deposited deep inside women. During arousal lubricating fluid may appear at the tip of the penis and this contains some sperms. Most of the sperms, of course, are released when the man ejaculates or climaxes. After intercourse the penis returns to its normal size, which is smaller than during the excited state. This is why contraceptive sheaths need to be removed as soon as sex is over, because the sudden change in size can lead to leakage of sperms from the side of the sheath, and the risk of pregnancy.

2

Contraception

In the last chapter we discussed the ways in which a pregnancy could start. The rest of the book is about stopping pregnancies, but first we should ask why this is necessary. It is important to remember that throughout human history some form of contraception has been used, with most sexual activity being for recreation rather than procreation. Most pairs in the animal kingdom produce in their turn only two further offspring who are capable of breeding. This is just as true for humans as for starlings who lay 16 eggs in their lifetime and codfish who lay 40 million. The important difference is that while codfish rely on massive wastage of eggs, and earlier human societies relied on high infant mortality rates coupled with not very effective natural methods, people today are unwilling to accept wasted pregnancies. They demand that the methods they use to prevent unplanned pregnancies be reliable, safe, and easy to use.

Humans have existed on earth for about five million years. For all but the last thousand most women spent much of their adult reproductive life either pregnant or breast-feeding. This happens in very few societies today, and in the West women generally expect to have started a career, or at least had a few years of freedom, before their first pregnancy. In the years between puberty and first baby they need good contraception, as much for socio-economic reasons as for beliefs in personal freedom.

Human fertility

Despite our concern over population, the human race is not a particularly fertile one. Farmers, who admittedly use strains of animals bred for high fertility, expect most of their animals to have at least one offspring as a result of one mating; in human societies this is the exception rather than the rule. Although records are poor, it seems that fecundability rates, which are the likelihood of a baby occurring after a single act of intercourse, are as low now in Western Europe as they have been for the last 200 years. They vary according to the age of the woman, with a peak between the ages of 20 and 30, but even at their highest are only 25 per cent or so. To put it more simply, if a fertile couple have intercourse with no contraception on the most fertile day possible, the woman has a one in four chance of a baby (the chances of starting a pregnancy are, of course, a bit higher as not all pregnancies come to term). This means that three times out of four intercourse, even without contraception, will fail to produce a baby. (This might seem a rather boring statistical concept but it is important in understanding contraceptive effectiveness rates.)

How effective is contraception?

To simplify discussion, most contraceptives are quoted as failing x number of times in 100 woman-years of use. This ignores the fact that all methods of contraception are more effective in older women and those who have never had children (because about 10 per cent of women who have never had children will be unable to have them for reasons other than their use of contraception). It also implies that we can study 100 women using a method for a year and expect the same results as 10 women using a method for 10 years, or any other sort of permutation of numbers of women and years. This method of calculation takes no account of side-effects, or the liking of the couple for the method; and perhaps one of its biggest disadvantages is that it does not readily distinguish between failures due to the method not

Contraception

working and failures due to the couple not using the method—which can often be related to side-effects.

The likeliest time for failures to occur is during the first year of use. This is because some couples will still be practising with their method, and methods like the cap.need much practice to ensure their reliability. Some of the women who get pregnant in the first few months of contraceptive use will be those who are very fertile, or those who were not keen on using any method of contraception; while those who use a method successfully for many years with no problems will be a mixture of the lucky, the relatively subfertile, and those who are strongly motivated not to become pregnant. They will of course also be many years older on average!

The methods available for any particular couple will depend on many factors. It may not even be the couple who make the decision but just one of the partners—usually the woman. The aim of this book is to give the facts, while those concerned must make up their own minds. In Chapter 13 we discuss some of the cultural influences on contraception, but there are other factors that affect the availability of contraceptive services. Such factors include religious pressures acting through the State. In Eire almost all contraceptive methods are not widely available. Some Third World countries, like Malawi, restrict the availability of contraception even more thoroughly. Japan is a developed country where many Western methods of contraception are unavailable or discouraged. This is because for many years abortion was one of the more important methods of birth control and the medical profession, who had a lucrative hold on abortion services, fought against the introduction of any method that might interfere with their profit-making. In Sweden, where contraception is taught openly in schools and abortion in early pregnancy is freely available on request, vasectomy is infrequently offered and is still of doubtful legality. The excuse given by Swedish family planners is that the shadow of the Nazi holocaust with its forced eugenic sterilizations has been a long time settling.

Changes in contraception

One of the more important changes to occur in contraceptive practice over the past four decades has been the change in acceptability of the subject. A book such as this would have been unthinkable 20 years ago, as well as being impossible (from the point of view of the methods described) 30 years ago. When Marie Stopes first published *Married Love* in 1923 it was considered pornographic. Many family-planning doctors can still remember the bitter debates provoked by the proposal to provide contraception to the unmarried. Some of us can remember our teachers at medical school emphasizing that the pill was suitable for only a few married women who had completed their families! There are still clinics in some parts of Britain which demand written consent from a woman's husband before fitting an IUCD, but they are becoming fewer as the right of women to decide on their own contraception becomes more established. We have come a long way but there is still much to be done.

An example of the changes occurring is one of the United Kingdom government surveys published in 1979. This was carried out by the government offices dealing with censuses, and was the first ever government survey conducted in Britain which asked all those women interviewed about their contraceptive usage. The survey (Karen Dunnell: *Family formation 1976*; Office of Population Censuses and Surveys (1979)) not only studied contraceptive use by single and formerly married women, but also asked married women about their use of contraceptives before marriage.

The figures are extremely detailed and those who are interested can read the original publication. The important points were that 72 per cent of all women aged between 16 and 49 were using a contraceptive method at the time of interview. (Two-thirds of the remainder were not in a sexual relationship at that time, which means that almost all women who were sexually active were using contraception.)

The most commonly used method was the pill, with 28 per cent of all women using it, or 39 per cent of all those using contraception. This was naturally dependent on their age, with 54 per cent of those between 20 and 24 taking the pill, and only 8 per cent of those between 45 and 49. The next most common method was the sheath, with 16 per cent of all women using it, and 28 per cent in the older age range.

All other methods were uncommon. Seven per cent of women had been sterilized, and 6 per cent were relying on their sterilized partners. Another 6 per cent (mainly older women) were relying on coitus interruptus, while 5 per cent used the IUCD. Two per cent were using the cap and all other methods (principally the natural ones) accounted for a further 2 per cent.

Another interesting survey on contraceptive usage came from the University of Oxford. Researchers there studied over 4000 women who stopped using contraception in order to have a baby. These were almost equally divided between women who had used the pill and those who were using other methods, principally the barriers. Only 266 out of the 4356 had used the IUCD. The most reassuring finding was that all the women seemed to get pregnant at about the same sort of rate. Many of the women who stopped using the pill took an extra few months to return to normal fertility, but no group had any evidence of long-term impairment of fertility.

The next chapter is going to discuss one of the most popular methods of all time, the oral contraceptive pill. The generation since it arrived has seen dramatic changes in public attitudes to contraception, and the pill has played a large part in this.

11

3

The pill

Introduction

At the present time more women use the pill than any other method of contraception in the United Kingdom, and in certain groups of women more are using it than all other methods put together. This is particularly true of young women between 20 and 25 years of age. Probably the best indicator of its acceptance is the fact that we no longer use a capital P or inverted commas when writing about it—everyone understands that 'the pill' refers only to one kind of tablet! There has been more research about the pill, and more written about it, than almost any other drug. It has been blamed for social revolution and the spread of everything from women's liberation to venereal disease.

This chapter is about the combined (two-hormone) oral contraceptive, the method we normally mean when talking about the pill. There is another form of contraception which uses only one hormone. This is sometimes called the 'mini-pill', which is a confusing title because almost all of the oral contraceptive tablets now in use are 'mini' in the sense that they are low in hormone dosage. This second group of pills use only chemicals that are broken down in the body to give compounds that act like progesterone, and so they are more usually called progestogen-only pills. They will be dealt with in the next chapter.

Oral contraception has been a dream of humanity for many centuries. Most societies have traditions of medicines that, when swallowed, will prevent pregnancy. Some of them undoubtedly produced abortions, but the dream of something simple and easy to take has been with us for a long time. One of the earliest records of a preparation for

The pill

preventing pregnancy is in an ancient Chinese text, which recommended swallowing 24 live tadpoles. If these were swallowed in spring the woman concerned could look forward to five years of freedom from pregnancy. Albert the Great in the Middle Ages suggested that bees rather than tadpoles should be eaten.

Modern oral contraception began in the late 1940s with the discovery that the roots of the wild Mexican yam could produce the basic ingredient for many of the steroid hormones which are present in the body. (In fact, one of the first companies to market oral contraceptives, Syntex, derived its name from *synt*hesis and *Mex*ico.) It had been known for some decades that giving pure hormones to women and female animals affected ovulation but, because natural hormones are very expensive and rapidly broken down in the digestive system, the new findings were a breakthrough. Until then the only source of hormones was from animals. For example one laboratory used four tons of sows' ovaries to isolate just 25 mg of pure oestrogen. For the first time large quantities of hormones could be prepared in the laboratory, cheaply and quickly, and their molecules rearranged in such a way that the derivatives would be active when taken by mouth, but still act as pure hormones in the body.

The first women to try the new tablets lived in Boston and clinical trials were then started in Puerto Rico. The early pills had great quantities of drugs compared with the much smaller dosages in use today, but they filled a need. Within 20 years their use had spread across the globe, with about 60 million women around the world using them now.

Interestingly enough, the early development of the pill was paid for and inspired by American feminists. They saw it as the long-awaited answer to the problem of unwanted pregnancy, and they stepped in where pharmaceutical companies feared to tread. Most of the big drug companies, especially in the United States, were afraid that if they too openly espoused chemicals like these they might precipitate a consumer boycott of their other products! Professor Robert Greenblatt tells the story of the first time that he heard about the new drugs. He was at a hormone conference, at which the inventors presented their work. They showed that women who took these drugs had their ovulation suppressed. Professor Greenblatt stood up and proclaimed that they had 'unwittingly given us an excellent oral contraceptive'. Both Drs Rock and Pincus, who had presented the work with Dr C. R. Garcia, came up to him afterwards and begged him never to use the word contraceptive again—it would cause them too many problems if the press thought that their research involved contraception!

During the decade following the first use of the pill changes occurred, but very few of them were in the actual chemicals involved. Several of the hormones which are now used were among the first to be synthesized, and the only major changes have been in the dosages used. The biggest change has been in the receptiveness of the population to the drugs. There was once an overwhelming desire to see every woman take the pill, and it was seen as the answer to almost every fertility and gynaecological problem. The first big scare was the publication in 1968 of studies that showed a significant link between the use of oral contraceptives and thrombosis (blood clots) in the veins. This had first been hinted at in 1961 but definitive studies were a long time in coming. It was some time before it was realized that more than oestrogens are linked with blood-clotting, there are other factors as well. Obesity and a sedentary way of life are just as important, and, possibly even more important, are factors in the family history which predispose to these conditions. Many authorities feel that cigarette smoking is the most important single factor for developing blood clots in arteries, but not in veins.

These problems provoked a backlash and throughout the world many hundreds of thousands of women stopped taking the pill they had come to rely on. There were many unwanted pregnancies, but at the same time careful epidemiological research helped to bring about a more balanced view of the pill. Doctors began to realize that it is the safest form of contraception for young, healthy women, while the risks probably outweighed the benefits for older women with risk factors like high blood pressure. Most women are in between the two ends of the spectrum, and we hope that this chapter will help them to decide if the potential risks outweigh the benefits for them.

The main use for the pill is of course to provide a safe and efficient means of contraception, but it also has other uses. It can be used as an emergency method for after-sex birth control when a risk has been taken (see Chapter 8). It can also be used to treat period problems, and sometimes as a medicine in its own right to treat diseases like endometriosis. We will discuss these other uses after we have discussed the main use for the pill which is to provide simple, easy, efficient, and reversible contraception.

Types of pill

The pill is a mixture of two main types of hormone, one that mimics progesterone and the other a derivative of oes-trogen. There are only two types of oestrogen used in the pill, ethinyl oestradiol and one of its derivatives, mestranol. There are several different progestogens, with norgestrel and norethisterone being the two main ones and accounting for about nine-tenths of all oral contraceptives sold in the United Kingdom (norgestrel pills alone account for 80 per cent).

The dosage of oestrogen is fairly constant. Because of the links between oestrogen and blood-clotting, and because other side-effects tend to be related to the dose of oestrogen, the trend over the past few years has been to lower the oestrogen dose in each pill. The commonest tablets now in use have only 30 millionths of a gram of oestrogen, which is about one-seventh of the dose that the earliest volunteers were given. There is very little difference between the two varieties of oestrogen, which is hardly surprising as mestranol is mainly converted to ethinyl oestradiol in the body.

The progestogens show a much greater variability in dose and type. A large part of the reason for this is commercial as some of the progestogens are marketed by one company only, while oestrogens are much more widely available.

There is no such thing as the 'best pill', though nearly all doctors agree that the aim should be to give the lowest possible dose of both the hormones. Most will routinely prescribe one of the standard pills with a maximum of 30 or 35 micrograms of oestrogen. The particular brand of pill used is largely immaterial, and most doctors will prescribe the one that they have found in the past to be the most suitable. For most women the pill that suits them is the same one that might suit their sisters or next-door neighbours.

A recent study carried out by the World Health Organization compared six different types of pill and found almost no differences between any of them. All the pills were low in hormone content, and neither the women nor the doctors doing the testing in centres around the world were told at the time which type of pill they were using. The differences between the acceptability of the different pills were slight, with the only really important findings being that the pill with only 20 micrograms of oestrogen caused more accidental pregnancies amongst its users and apparently also more bleeding problems—mostly extra bleeding between periods.

Probably the most worrying feature was that pregnancy rates (which were between 1 and 6 per cent depending on the centre involved) were higher than we have come to expect for the pill. It is possible that the way the trial was carried out made failure more likely, or it could be that in our efforts to lower pill dosage we are now so close to the limits of effectiveness that some women are teetering on the brink of pregnancy each month. An interesting fact is that of the 72 unplanned pregnancies 38 were from India. Some people have put forward the argument that Indian women living in India on traditional Indian diets may respond to steroid hormones in a different way to Western women. In several comparative trials from organizations like the World Health Organization, where the same drug has been given to women in many different parts of the world, there have been higher failure rates in the Indian section of the experiment.

How the pill works

The pill acts mainly by preventing the release of an egg from the ovary. Development of the next egg to be released starts before menstruation, when all of the hormones involved are at a very low level. This low level triggers off the release of a hormone from the pituitary gland (*F*ollicle *S*timulating *H*ormone or FSH) which starts the final development of as many as 40 eggs. One, or sometimes more, of these eggs become dominant and the release of the dominant egg is triggered by a sudden surge of *L*uteinizing *H*ormone (LH). This sudden surge has itself been triggered off by the increasing amount of oestrogen produced by the growing follicle containing the soon-to-be-released egg.

The pill provides a steady hormone level that prevents the interplay of hormones and so stops ovulation. The absence of ovulation also means an absence of the hormonal changes that accompany it. While some of these—for example, the premenstrual syndrome—are not directly related to fertility, others are. The hormones from the developing follicle stimulate the cervix, or neck of the womb, to produce the mucus needed for the safe conduct of sperm. These hormones also prepare the lining of the womb to accept the fertilized egg. These effects are modified in women on the pill. They are important additional effects, because some women ovulate intermittently while on the pill. This is particularly likely to happen if they are taking their pills erratically, especially if they are on the low-dose pills. Since this might lead to pregnancy a back-up system is needed, and the other actions of the pill provide this—they make the system inhospitable to sperms and they prevent the implantation of fertilized eggs.

How to take the pill

There are four different types of pill, and so four different sets of rules for taking them. They all have one thing in common—the pills function best when taken regularly, and preferably at the same time of day or night.

The commonest type of pill is the 21-, or occasionally 22-day pack. All of the tablets are the same and each tablet is in a separate blister in the packet. Each blister is labelled consecutively and has a day of the week printed on it. On the first day that a pill is taken one is chosen from a blister marked for that particular day of the week, and the pills are then taken one after the other every day until the packet is finished. On the 22-day packets the last pill is taken on the same day of the week that the packet was started. The most commonly used packs are the 21-day ones, and the last pill in these packets is taken on the day of the week before the day that the pack was first started.

There are also other types of pill packet. Less common now than they once were are the 28-day packets. These were a variation on the 21-day packets but with an additional seven 'blank' tablets. The idea was that some women might get out of the habit of swallowing tablets if they had to have a whole week away from them and so, rather than miss any days out, seven hormone-free tablets were included. This seemed a good idea at the time but is only popular in a few parts of the world, like Australia and New Zealand.

The new variable dose pills are more complicated. These

The pill

are relatively new in family planning use, although the hormones which they use are in fact the usual ones. They have both hormones in every pill but the relative amounts differ. There are two main types of this pill—those with three different levels of hormone (the triphasic pills) and those with only two (the biphasic pills). Just to complicate the issue, while most of them are 21-day packets, one of the triphasic preparations (Logynon-ED) is a 28-day version of Logynon with seven blank tablets.

The triphasic preparations were launched on to the United Kingdom market in 1980, although they had been used in continental Europe for some while before that. There are three different levels of hormone in them, with an increasing level of hormone as the month progresses. The reasoning behind this is a mixture of wanting to 'mimic' the normal cycle and to provide the lowest possible overall hormone dosage, while giving the largest dose at the time when it is most needed. The biphasic preparation is similar and newer. There are two levels of hormones and the dose of these increases as the month advances.

All of these tablets are only effective if they are taken regularly. Obviously, this does not always happen and we need to consider some of the effects of missing pills. This can happen when the woman accidentally forgets to take a pill or when she does take the pill but something happens to stop it being absorbed. The latter usually happens through interaction with other drugs, or because of diarrhoea or vomiting.

When to start the course

One point that should be discussed is the best time to start taking the pill. There are many old wives' tales about this, with several books advocating unnecessary delay. For instance, after the end of a pregnancy there is no real need to wait for the first period before resuming the pill—it is perfectly possible to start straight away, or at least within a few days. Although it may be theoretically safer to wait until the baby is four weeks old, starting the pill straight away has the advantage of getting you into a routine. While pregnancy is extremely unlikely in the first few weeks after a baby has been born, there is no real need to take unnecessary chances. Some people worry that since both the pill and pregnancy can predispose to blood-clotting problems, taking the pill immediately after pregnancy doubles the risk. But the hormone content of the pill is so small when compared with the hormone levels produced in pregnancy that it is not really dangerous.

When the first pills came on to the market it was felt that they should be taken around the end of a period. To produce some sort of standardization the fifth day from the start of the period was taken as the day on which to start the pills, and they were then taken for the next 21 days. The proviso was also made that they would not be effective for the first month, and so some other form of contraception was needed. Most doctors now say that starting on the first day of the period is not only much easier but will also provide instant contraception. There is a disadvantage of course—in the first month of using them there is more bleeding and spotting. Most women find this a small price to pay as long as they know beforehand that this will happen.

What to do if a tablet is forgotten

With the best will in the world tablets do get forgotten, or are taken during periods of illness when they might be vomited up, or hurried through the intestine before being absorbed. Obviously, that day's tablet is lost forever, but what is the correct thing to do? Authorities still argue about this, and the best thing we can do is to set out the facts and let the people who will carry the burden of pregnancy make up their own minds.

Everybody agrees that if one pill is forgotten, and the

mistake is realized within a few hours—say, 12—the best thing to do is to take the missed pill then and the next one at the usual time. This sort of accident is common and while it should not become a habit does not usually lead to pregnancy or any other problems.

Much more debatable though is what action to take when there is a longer gap between taking pills. The pill manufacturers say that if the gap is 36 hours or more then the two missing pills should be taken together, and some other form of contraception taken for the rest of the packet. This is probably safe, but ignores the fact that the risk of pregnancy can be greatest some days after the accident rather than at the time it happens. This is because the pill acts by 'switching-off' that part of the hypothalamus that controls ovulation, and if this becomes active again it can lead to the release of the hormones which will start the production of another egg. This egg may be released seven or more days later, so it is best to assume that some form of contraception other than the pill is needed for the next 14 days. This is still true even if the next 14 days include a period, and the first few days after it.

Many drugs interact with the pill. While some of these are rather obscure antibiotics used for the treatment of tuberculosis or leprosy, others are common, important, and used for treating diseases like bronchitis, tonsillitis, and cystitis. Ampicillin is one of these drugs, and if your doctor starts you on Penbritin or ampicillin remember to use an additional method of contraception for at least the rest of that cycle and the first week of the next one if you are taking ampicillin near the end of a packet. All doctors should tell patients who get prescriptions about the side-effects of the drugs they are prescribing and about the interactions of those drugs with the pill, or alcohol, or similar things. If your doctor does prescribe any medicines for you it is worth reminding him that you are on the pill and ask if there is an interaction. This does not only apply to antibiotics, but to a number of other common medicines, like those used for treating epilepsy. There are few good reasons for stopping the pill unless the woman herself wants to. Many years ago it was taught that people taking the pill should have a two-month break from it every year or two to let the hormones be removed from their body. Recent research has not shown any important effect of duration of use, and most authorities feel that if someone is happy on the pill then she should continue with it until she wants to become pregnant, or wishes to change to another method of contraception.

Pregnancy during pill taking

Something which worries many of the people involved in contraceptive research is the effect of the pill on the pregnancies that might occur after a few pills have been forgotten. As a general rule, pregnancies occurring after the pill has been stopped are the same as any other. The University of Oxford/Family Planning Association study that we discussed in Chapter 2 showed that women who stopped using the pill to become pregnant were just as fertile as their counterparts who had been using other methods of contraception. The only difference was that many of the women who stopped the pill had a delayed return of fertility for a few months. There seemed to be no difference in the rate at which they lost those pregnancies, or in the defects that their children had, or even in the sex of the children.

However, it is women who conceive while taking the pill, or possibly in the first few weeks after stopping it, who present a more complex picture. This is partly because many of these pregnancies are unwanted, and so end up as abortions, and also because many other factors influence the outcome of the pregnancy. Because the variables range from maternal age and social class through racial grouping to things like cigarette and alcohol consumption, there are few studies that have been done which take every possible good or adverse effect on pregnancy into consideration.

Two main trends seem to be emerging from the literature, however. Women who conceive while they are still taking the pill may have an increased risk of a baby with an excessively rare condition, namely, 'limb reduction defect'. In this condition the arms and legs are either absent or shortened. Despite the fact that many women have become pregnant while they were taking the pill (and it has been suggested that there are 70 000 such pregnancies each year in the USA), most doctors working in the field of child health have never seen a single infant with these abnormalities. Since 1 in 50 babies is born with some significant abnormality, this minute added risk should not alter what you decide to do about a pregnancy. The other interesting trend is that there might be a slightly increased likelihood of babies born after oral contraceptive failure being boys. This might also be true of pregnancies occurring a few weeks after the pill has been stopped, but it is difficult to be sure of this.

Positive reasons for using the pill

There are some women for whom the pill is the best method of contraception, and it is so ideally suited to them that there need to be very strong reasons for anything else to be chosen in preference. This does not mean of course that they have no choice in the matter—only that clinical experience involving many women has suggested that for these women the pill is the most suitable method of contraception.

The pill is very often the best method of contraception for couples who have a sexual difficulty. Because it provides almost complete freedom from fear of pregnancy, one more potential barrier to sexual enjoyment is removed. The use of the pill is not directly related to intercourse, and so there is no interruption of the normal flow of events from first sexual arousal to intercourse. Neither does it require the woman to examine herself or be examined regularly at a clinic, which most women can tolerate but some find acutely distressing. It also tends not to cause inter-menstrual bleeding or prolonged periods, which can be disconcerting to some couples. Some men find the use of condoms an embarrassing experience. They sometimes lose their erections, or even ejaculate, while putting them on. Others find that condom use leads to worries and makes them self-conscious about the size of their penis or their sexual performance.

Another group of women who are probably well-suited to the pill, but about whom there are more arguments, are those who are confined to a wheel-chair. While there is no reason for these women not to have babies, they often worry more about unplanned pregnancies than their more active counterparts. They find longer periods and inter-menstrual spotting are more of a problem because sanitary protection is much harder to organize from the confines of a wheel-chair. Similarly, the ease with which other women can walk to the bathroom and pop in a diaphragm does not apply to them. For them a pill that might shorten, or even suppress, periods is a boon. One worry is the fact that they might be more prone to developing blood clots in their legs. This is because one of the factors that makes blood clots more likely is lack of movement, and some people believe that the arteries and veins of paralyzed legs are more likely to develop blood clots. Experience with many women who have taken the pill suggests that this does not seem to be a problem, and if the risk is explained to them many will be prepared to take it.

Another group of women who might benefit more from the pill than any other form of contraception is the young. In Chapter 6 we discuss the benefits of barrier methods for this group, but there is a stronger case for the pill. It is reliable and can also control the period irregularities and painful periods that afflict many young girls. There is also some evidence that it can reduce the incidence of pelvic infections which they might develop, unlike the IUCD which might actually increase the likelihood of these infections.

We have talked a lot about the snags of the pill, but it is important to remember that the pill offers a number of health advantages besides protection from unwanted pregnancy.

The changes that the pill produces in cervical mucus give some protection against infection within the womb and the Fallopian tubes, though the sheath and the cap provide even better protection.

The pill also protects against both cancer of the ovary and of the endometrium. These cancers are only half as common in pill users as in those who have not used it, and in the case of cancer of the endometrium the benefits from taking the pill seem to last for at least ten years after the pill has been stopped.

As we have said the situation regarding breast cancer is uncertain for high dose pills in younger women, while in those over the age of 25 there seems to be no effect. Benign (non-cancerous) lumps in the breast are much less common in pill users.

The other benefits of the pill have been implied in what we have already said. Because of the lighter periods which the pill gives, heavy periods and subsequent anaemia are prevented. Painful periods in young women seem only to occur in months when an egg is released, and so, because it prevents ovulation, the pill cures this problem better than any other treatment. A number of other conditions may be improved. Headaches often get better. Teenage spots (acne) get better, especially with the triphasic pill. Premenstrual symptoms get better in a quarter of all women, while taking the pill continously (without the 'week off' between packets) will help most women with premenstrual tension.

Because the pill protects against pelvic infections and

stops ovulation, ectopic pregnancy (pregnancy outside the womb) is very rare in women who use the pill. This form of pregnancy is uncommon, but can be dangerous.

Reasons for not using the pill

The pill is not the best answer for everyone. There are some women who should probably never use it, and others who should only use it with care, once they have had the opportunity to read and weigh the evidence. Among those unsuited to the pill are women who are likely to develop severe vascular disease. These women include those who smoke or have had vascular disease in the past, or have high blood pressure. One of the biggest risk factors is family tendency to this sort of disease, and most authorities would say that if a woman has relatives who have suffered from severe disease of the heart and blood-vessels, like heart attacks, very early in life, then it is probably best for her not to take the pill, and she should also seek specialist advice. This really only applies to women who have had close relatives who had severe disease while still in their thirties. There is also some evidence to suggest that women who smoke cigarettes have a particularly high rate of blood-vessel disease while taking the pill. This is much higher in them than it is in those who just smoke or just take the pill, which suggests that the two habits act together to increase the amount of damage that the blood-vessel walls suffer.

Women with diabetes fall into a special group. The pill alters the way in which their bodies handle sugar but the change, once it has occurred, is constant. Once they are well established on the pill their insulin requirements are not going to change very much. This means that although there is a definite change after they have started the pill it remains steady and so can be accounted for. Many doctors worry that since both diabetes and the pill have been linked with disease of the blood-vessels, the two together might cause more severe disease to occur sooner. Like many stories about the risks of taking the pill it is not easy to prove this one, but most doctors now feel that the low-dose pill is safer for diabetic women than the risks of pregnancy.

A problem occurs with women who have sickle-cell anaemia. This is a disease that is found almost exclusively in black people. A defect in the production of the red blood pigment, haemoglobin, makes these people prone to produce sickle-shaped red blood cells, which clog up small blood-vessels and can lead to the formation of blood clots. If they are not looked after carefully, many of these people die young. Even with the best possible medical care they have many health problems and pregnancy poses many difficulties. While very few now die in pregnancy, this is more of a tribute to the skills of their medical attendants than good luck. More so for them than for other women, unplanned pregnancies are best avoided. The pill is an extremely good way of doing this, even though it too may predispose to blood clots. These women face so many problems with pregnancy and contraception that some doctors argue that, to be absolutely safe, they should avoid all sexual experience until they want children, and then complete their family while they are still young and healthy. They should use the pill for spacing their childbearing and then be sterilized. This would cut down the amount of time that they are exposed to any risk from contraception. In fact progestogen-only injections seem to be the safest method of contraception for sickle-cell sufferers, but this method may not be acceptable for everybody.

Side-effects

There are a great many side-effects attributable to the pill. Some of these are major, and important, while others are probably of little importance. The effect on the blood-vessels and the heart is important and serious, although thankfully uncommon. Very common, and probably of little importance, is the fact that less ear wax is produced in women who take the pill. They tend to go to their doctors less often to have their ears syringed. Pill side-effects can be divided into two main groups—those which might be related to the oestrogen part of the pill, and those which might be related to the progestogen component. Because the two hormones interact it is not easy in practice to distinguish the effect of the one from that of the other.

The side-effects from oestrogen are related to the amount in the pill and so they are less severe and less frequent in low dose preparations. They include headaches, dizziness, nausea, and water retention. Water retention leads to weight gain and a feeling of bloatedness, and might be linked with a rise in blood pressure and an increase in the size of the breasts. Other side-effects include an increase in vaginal mucus discharge, a decrease in milk flow in some breast-feeding women, and leg aches and pains, especially in women who have varicose veins. These leg pains are not the precursors of blood clots in the legs, or even any particular sign of disease, but they may bother women who have them and they often worry their doctors as well. The best policy is to treat the varicose veins or, if possible, live with the pain, but most women are happy with either a lower dose pill or, more usually, a different method of contraception.

The pill also affects the liver. Most women have a change in the composition of their bile, leading to an increase in the incidence of gall-stones, though since this only occurs in the early years of pill use it suggests that the pill is accelerating rather than causing the problem. Very rarely some women get an intensely itchy form of jaundice, rather like the jaundice that these women may suffer from in pregnancy. A few women develop benign tumours of the liver—but these are extremely rare.

The most serious side-effect of oestrogens is on blood clotting. They make blood much more likely to clot, and the clots can occur very suddenly in blood-vessels. If they are only in small blood-vessels in the back of the calf then, by themselves, they will not do much harm. The worry is though that not only can these blood-vessels be damaged for ever, but the blood clots can spread and involve the lungs. They can also occur in the brain, and even a small clot here can be fatal or extremely disabling. This side-effect is extremely rare and, now that very few women take more than 35 micrograms of ethinyl oestradiol a day, rarer still than it was 15 years ago.

It is much harder to distinguish the progestogen side-effects. This is because there are many different prog-estogens, with differing doses and potencies, and there is not the clear relationship between drug and side-effect which is found with oestrogens. The progestogens are said to predispose to long-term weight gain (as opposed to the rapid short-term weight gain of the oestrogens), tiredness, depression, and a decrease in sexual drive and feelings. They are also said to make greasy skin problems more likely and to produce a relative dryness in the vagina.

Migraine

Some women find that when taking the pill their migraine headaches get better, but for some they get worse. Mig-raines are very unpleasant, and so, in general, if the pill is making them worse, it is better not to take it. You should also stop the pill if migraine appears for the first ever time, or changes its character. This is particularly true of focal migraine.

Focal migraine is a form of migraine in which the symptoms are much more clearly defined than is usual in this condition. Instead of the numbing, crushing, pounding headache there is a much more localized pain, and it may be followed by, or happen at the same time as, a sign that the blood flow to part of the brain has been temporarily slowed down. These signs include: a sudden onset of temporary but profound tingling or weakness of part of the body (perhaps the whole of one side, or just part of the arm); the loss of part of your field of vision; difficulty in speaking; an epileptic fit; or even sudden unconsciousness.

All of these symptoms are extremely rare, but they could be a sign of reduced blood flow to the brain. If they occur, then stop taking the pill and telephone your doctor immediately. You will not come to any harm, but your doctor will probably suggest that you never take the pill again.

Cancer

The most feared, and talked about, side-effect of the pill probably does not exist. Some years ago Professor Roger Short was asked to conduct a seminar on contraception with Honours students on a Zoology degree course in Edinburgh. The first question he asked was about the side-effects of the pill and there was an almost unanimous belief that the only important side-effect was cancer! This was from a population of students many of whom were probably already taking the pill. We shall devote several pages to the pill and cancer. In general, most cancers have no effect on the pill and it has no effect on them. There are some cancers which if actually present are 'hormone-dependent'. This means that to grow they need to be stimulated by hormones. Some types of womb and breast cancer fall into this group. Here again there is the problem of pregnancy being a much bigger source of a hormonal stimulus than the pill; most women will probably produce fewer hormones if they take the pill than if they use another method and ovulate, or conceive, normally. Caution dictates that women who actually have oestrogen-sensitive cancers should not use the pill.

There is no conclusive evidence linking the pill as a causative agent with any form of cancer. It is true that the induction period of most cancers is long—of the order of 15 years or more—but the pill has been around for longer.

The pill

While there are very few women who have been taking the pill for that length of time, there are so many women taking it that any trends should have become apparent by now. They have not.

Breast cancer is the commonest type of cancer afflicting women in the Western world. The cause for it is not yet known, but hormonal influences are almost certainly involved. Some authorities feel that one of the factors responsible for the fact that there is more breast cancer in the West than in the Third World is that Western women delay their first pregnancy for many years. Women in the Third World are more likely to become pregnant at a younger age, and more often, and breast-feed, than their Western counterparts. Since the pill is part of the way in which women can delay childbirth, it is inevitable that some day a link will be found between the pill and breast cancer. It might well be that the decision to delay childbirth, and not the way in which it is done, is the more important factor.

Since 1981 there have been five large studies that have tried to discover possible links between the pill and cancer of the breast. All of these studies have been reassuring, suggesting that there does not seem to be any association, even after many years of use. However, in late 1983, Professor Malcolm Pike, who had been working in Los Angeles, published some new research. He suggested that there may be a link between the use of high dose pills for long periods of time by young women and later development of breast cancer. Fortunately, nearly all of the pills in his 'dangerous' group are no longer on the market, and few of them were ever given to young users anyway. However, one or two of the brands that were implicated in Professor Pike's study are widely used and, until more evidence is available, women who plan to have more than six years without a break on the pill before they reach the age of 25 should seek advice from their doctors on the most appropriate brand of pill for them. In general, this means following our usual rule, and using the lowest dose of oestrogen and progestogen that suits them.

One cancer which might be on the increase, again for reasons linked with but not caused by the pill, is cancer of the cervix (the neck of the womb). Again, nobody knows the cause of this cancer but it is linked (somehow) with sexual intercourse and might be related to a cancer-causing agent carried by men. Women nowadays tend to be more sexually active than once was the case, for which the pill might be in part responsible, and they also use barrier methods of contraception much less frequently. The convenience of the pill is to blame for this. Using the pill does not make women more likely to get cervical cancer but does make it more likely that it will be detected sooner. This is because most women on the pill have regular cervical smears taken at the clinic or doctor's surgery where they collect their prescriptions for the pill. These smears will often show up changes at a pre-cancerous stage where it can be treated easily, often with no damage to the rest of the womb or the ovaries. An interesting aside is that one study showed that women who came to a clinic and requested the pill had a greater likelihood of having pre-cancerous changes in the cervix than those who asked for other methods!

There are two other important cancers in the genital tract which have definite links with the pill. Cancer of the main part of the womb (the uterus) is much less common in women who take the pill than in those who do not. A recent American study showed that it almost never occurred in women who had taken the pill for eight years or more. This might be because the progestogen contained in the pill is also used to treat this form of cancer. Since something similar to this cancer can be produced experimentally by giving oestrogens alone, and then removed by giving progestogens, this is probably a real link and not just a coincidence.

The pill also has a protective effect on ovarian cancer.

The pill

This is a relatively common cancer that is often not diagnosed until too late, because of the way in which the ovaries are buried deep within the rest of the body. It might be that many years of being 'switched-off' (by the pill) rather than on again/off again, makes cancer less likely to develop.

There are a few other conditions around which there is controversy. Malignant melanomata, or cancerous moles on the skin, are uncommon in relatively sun-free climates like that of the United Kingdom. These moles are possibly linked with hormones because they can sometimes be successfully treated with anti-hormone drugs, like tamoxifen, and there is some evidence that the change from ordinary to cancerous moles is enhanced by oestrogens. The whole question is still unsettled, however. Similarly, while there is a link between the pill and the (very rare) benign liver tumours, the association between the pill and liver cancer is very uncertain.

Future fertility

There is still one area where women are concerned about the pill and that is its effect on future fertility. We have already mentioned the Oxford survey, which showed that women stopping the pill had a possible delay of a few weeks in their return to normal fertility. This is probably of no long-term (or even short-term) significance. Similarly, the rebound increase in fertility which was thought to occur when the pill was stopped is also probably rare and insignificant. There is no doubt that some women who stop the pill stop having periods at the same time. When this was believed to be a disease it was called 'post-pill amenorrhoea'. Most endocrinologists now believe that the title was a mistake which lulled them into a false sense of security. The cessation of periods is a sign that some sort of a disturbance is present, and while this might be only weight change or depression, it can sometimes be more serious. In most of these women the lack of periods might have been noticed many months earlier if it had not been masked by the regular bleeding produced by stopping the pill for seven days in each 28. Recent studies have shown that if these women are properly investigated and treated their fertility is the same as that of the rest of the population. Ninety-nine per cent of women who stop using the pill are having normal, regular periods within six months (unless they are pregnant). If you are one of the 1 per cent who are not—take advice.

Other uses for the pill

Although most women use the pill for contraception it is sometimes used to treat irregular periods and other gynaecological problems. In some societies, where contraception is not permitted or is only available with difficulty, menstrual regulation is the only reason for prescribing the pill. It is surprising how common menstrual problems are in those countries! The pill is one of the best methods available for treating erratic periods, since it will produce regular cycles of bleeding, even if they are not true periods. Before your doctor treats you with the pill for this reason, if you are over the age of 30 he will want to make sure that there is no underlying disease producing these symptoms. This usually involves sampling a small fragment of the womb lining (the endometrium) and sending it to a pathologist to be examined under the microscope. This procedure can be done in the clinic, but most British doctors prefer to do it in hospital under an anaesthetic. The procedure is known as a D & C (dilatation of the neck of the womb and curettage or scraping of the womb lining).

The pill can also be used to delay periods. This needs some forethought, and with the lower dose pills that are now in use it is not always as easy as it used to be. However, if someone is already taking the pill and wants to delay her next period, to avoid the inconvenience of having one when she is on holiday, or taking an examination, or getting married, then she need not wait seven days after finishing one packet before starting the next. Going straight from one packet to the next is easy and safe, and usually means that the next period will be delayed until the next seven-day break. A word of warning though—with the low-dose pills that are now almost standard many women find that extra days of bleeding become a problem. It is not as simple to take pills continuously when using the new triphasic or biphasic pills. The solution here is to take only the last row of pills—this unfortunately leaves many half-used packets which are of little use to anyone.

Some people worry about the extra dose of hormones taken when regularly using this method. This is understandable since, for an extra week of each month, tablets are being taken when once they were not, but this does not add up to very much—particularly when you remember that the hormone dosages in today's pills are about a third to a half of what they were ten years ago.

One disease that almost disappears during pill-taking is dysmenorrhoea (painful periods). Nobody knows the reason for the pain, but when ovulation is stopped by taking the pill then periods become less painful.

The premenstrual syndrome is a condition which affects a great many women, sometimes slightly but sometimes it can be disabling. It can be helped by taking the pill, although sadly the lower dose pills that we use today are less effective than the earlier higher dose pills. Some women find relief in taking the pill continuously. Instead of having a break of seven days every month they have one every few months, or maybe only once or twice a year. Surprisingly enough, in the first month that they do this they may still get the symptoms in the week before their period would have been due but not afterwards.

Some women who do not usually get premenstrual symptoms will develop them for the first time ever when they start low-dose pills, particularly the triphasic preparations. Nobody knows the real reason for this, but some of these women are helped by going onto higher-dose preparations. If they belong to that group of women who get depressed premenstrually, this can often get worse on the pill and they can end up depressed throughout the month.

Endometriosis is a rather unusual disease that is not fully understood. It is linked with pain in the pelvis and infertility, and most cases of it are discovered during investigations for infertility. Nobody knows how it begins but, when it is discovered, the picture is one of many of the cells that normally line the inside of the uterus (the endometrium) spreading over the inside of the abdomen. The patches of cells can be present as anything from a few discrete areas to large, blood-filled cysts that cause much pain and suffering. Treatment of the disease involves 'drying-up' the endometrium, and one of the most convenient ways of doing this is to use an oral contraceptive with a relatively high dose of a progestogen. This makes the endometrium shrink, both inside and outside the womb. If the pills are taken continuously there will be no periods, and so there will be no bleeding into the patches of endometriosis. This means that the cysts will stop growing and, as they shrink, the pain will get less.

Another condition that responds to the hormones in the pill is acne. Teenage acne is related to the hormonal changes that occur around the time of puberty, and one method of treatment which is not commonly used is the pill. The oestrogens present do seem to have a beneficial effect, although this is partially balanced by the progestogen component, and if a pill with a high progestogen content is taken the acne can get worse.

Summary

The pill acts mainly by preventing ovulation. It is widely used, and safe, and efficient, and reversible. It can harm the health of a few women and make life easier for many of the rest. It does not appear to cause cancers but might prevent some. There are some women for whom it is not suitable, especially the older smoker or the woman with blood pressure problems. The contraceptive that suits some of these women is another hormonal contraceptive—the progestogen-only one. It is similar to the pill we have talked about but can be taken either by mouth or given by injection.

4

Progestogen-only contraception

The combined (two-hormone) pill described in the previous chapter is the most widely used artificial contraceptive method in the world. The progestogen-only pill that we will describe in this chapter is used by only a minority of women, although it is in many ways similar to the combined pill.

Doctors involved in family planning work always say that progestogen-only contraception is A Good Thing, and most seem genuinely mystified when asked to explain its relative lack of popularity. One reason for this is the runaway success of the combined pill. This has resulted in inertia on the part of doctors. The first commercially available and acceptable contraceptive pill was the combined pill. Nobody wants to change a winning combination, and since the early reports on the progestogen-only pill emphasized its problems it failed to establish a niche.

Progestogen and progesterone

The progestogen-only pills are also known as the mini-pills but, as we discussed in the last chapter, this is an anachronistic and confusing term. They have only one chemical in them, which breaks down in the body to give progesterone-like compounds. Chemicals that do this are called progestogens, and throughout this book we will use the terms progestogen-only and progesterone-only contraception interchangeably. Progesterone itself, when given by mouth, is mostly digested before it can be absorbed into the bloodstream.

In contrast to the 40 or 50 different types of combined pills there are fewer than a dozen progestogen-only pills. Their share of the market is about 2 per cent of that of the other contraceptive pills. They use the same progestogens as the combined pills but in much smaller doses, and it is this fact that determines the way they are taken and their main side-effects.

How do the progestogen-only pills work?

These pills work in some ways like the combined pill. Sometimes they prevent ovulation, like the combined pill does, but their main method of action is to thicken up the cervical mucus and make the lining of the womb inhospitable to fertilized eggs. They almost certainly have an additional effect of making the Fallopian tubes contract less, which keeps any sperms that have penetrated the mucus from travelling along the tubes to the egg. It is also possible that they have a direct effect on the outer skin of sperms making them less able to fertilize eggs, and possibly a similar effect on the egg. Most of these other effects are small and secondary to the two main effects—that of thickening-up cervical mucus and changing the lining of the womb.

How to take the progesterone-only pill

The progestogen-only pill has to be taken every day. There is not a seven-days-off 21-days-on type of pattern. They need to be taken even during periods. Some of the manufacturers recommend that the pills should always be taken at about the same time of day, and suggest that they be taken at a time about four hours before intercourse is likely to occur. Their worry is that if the tablets are taken at bed-time, and intercourse takes place a few minutes later, the tablet will not have had time to be absorbed. This means that you will be depending for your protection on a pill taken 24 hours previously. The point of view has been put forward that the progestogen-only pills are more like a barrier method of contraception than a hormonal method, except that they take about three hours to be absorbed and become effective. If you do forget to take one at your usual time—take it as soon as possible. If you are more than three hours late in taking a pill, especially at mid-cycle, your protection will be reduced. If you have already had sex when you realize the problem, then post-coital contraception is a good idea—talk it over with your doctor.

Are they as effective as the combined pills?

Most textbooks say that this type of pill is less effective as a contraceptive than the standard version. Surprisingly enough, only once have researchers made a serious attempt to compare the effectiveness of the two different types at preventing pregnancy and they found very little difference. We mentioned in Chapter 2 that there are several ways of looking at contraceptive effectiveness rates. Bald figures are not enough; we need to try and define the type of population that is being studied and how well motivated the women are, as well as simple things like their age and previous fertility.

These pills need to be taken regularly and at about the same time of each day. They probably contain just enough hormone to be effective, and possibly for some women not quite enough. Many of the women taking this form of contraception are of the type we describe in Chapter 13 as 'spacers'—they are in between pregnancies and, no matter how highly motivated they may appear to be, they do in fact have higher pregnancy rates for almost every method of contraception. Since one of the biggest groups of women using progestogen-only contraception are 'spacers' these pills have been branded, probably unfairly, with the stigma of unreliability.

In a trial carried out by the World Health Organization that was published recently, women attending family planning clinics in two widely separated centres (one in India and the other in Yugoslavia) were given packets of pills in sealed

Progestogen-only contraception

envelopes. Half of the women were given combined pills while the other half were given progestogen-only pills. There were two kinds of each preparation and all four types were packed in 28-day packets (all of the combined-pill packets had seven blank tablets) so that nobody could tell which packet contained which type of drug. All of the women were told the nature of the experiment and that they should take a pill every day, whether they were having a period or not. When the results were analysed it was found that the two different types of progestogen-only pill were as effective at preventing pregnancy as one of the standard combined pills containing 50 μg of oestrogen. More effective than those three was one of the low-dose combined pills with only 30 μg of oestrogen! This experiment suggested that more important than the type of pill was the person taking it, and that there might be no significant difference between the two main types of pill.

This view clashes with orthodox medical opinion and with some of the experimental work carried out in other countries. Recently, for example, the University of Oxford/ Family Planning Association study published their work based on much larger groups of well-motivated women, and they showed that the failure rate for these preparations was almost ten times higher than for combined pills. Additional evidence for the fact that it is the population rather than the pill that is important comes from the large number of clinical trials from around the world which have shown great variations in the rates for almost every complication, from bleeding disturbances to pregnancy. Many of these studies quote rates for unplanned pregnancy that are the same as for the combined pill. Some in fact quoted rates for complications that were much higher than we have come to expect from combined pills. Pregnancy rates for the progestogen-only pill seem to be in the range of 0·5 to 4 for every hundred women using them for a year, compared with between 0·1 and 1 per cent for combined pills.

Side-effects

Bleeding

The commonest side-effect of this group of pills is an alteration of the normal bleeding pattern. Almost everyone who takes this pill says that their periods become irregular, with bleeding and spotting in between their periods, which may also change in character. A few people experience the reverse and develop longer gaps between their periods, with even fewer having no periods at all. This irregular bleeding can be difficult to control. If you take these pills you will still ovulate as you did before and so have periods as you did before. The tablets will often produce spotting of blood in between periods. One cynic has even suggested that these pills do not work at all—they just produce so much bleeding and spotting that couples stop having intercourse!

Most people find that the extra days of bleeding become fewer if they keep taking the tablets, with the first three months usually being the worst. Some women's periods stop altogether. Their biggest anxiety then is that they might have become pregnant. The best thing to do is to keep taking the tablets while a pregnancy is excluded. It is not easy to prove the presence of very early pregnancies and many people find the wait for proof so nerve-wracking that they eventually stop this type of pill to start using something else. If they do stay on this pill the absence of periods is a good sign. It implies that ovulation has been switched off by the prog-estogen-only pill. This makes it even more effective at stopping pregnancy and so, provided the woman's mind is set at rest from the fear of pregnancy, she will benefit more from this method of contraception than other women might.

Bleeding disturbances are the only real side-effect of the progestogen-only pill. One unfortunate consequence of the fact that they are prescribed much less frequently than the combined pills is that large-scale epidemiological surveys (which have been done on the combined pill) have not been possible. Most of the research done on these pills has been based on the experience of individual prescribers, or relatively small-scale but intensive studies on often remarkably few women. These studies have shown up few problems. These pills contain the same progestogens as the combined pill and have been available for about the same length of time.

Other side-effects

Careful experimental work has shown that, unlike the combined pill, progestogen-only pills do not increase the danger of blood-clotting to any significant degree; they do not seem to affect the way that the liver and thyroid work; and they do not increase blood pressure. It is possible that they might affect the handling of sugar in diabetics, but this danger is not as great as that of the combined pill. There is also no effect that we know of on breast-milk production, with very little of the hormone going through to the milk. In high doses over long periods of time they might alter the levels of fats in the bloodstream, and it has been suggested that this might predispose to disease of the blood-vessels. This is hypothesis rather than fact.

Complications of pregnancy

Women who have accidental pregnancies while taking the combined pill have the same risk of complications as any other pregnancy with possibly some added risk to the fetus (see p. 22). Pregnancies happening while taking the progestogen-only pill, though for the most part the same as those which occur on taking the combined pill, are said to have a much greater chance of being abnormally situated. These pregnancies are called ectopic pregnancies.

Ectopic pregnancy is in many ways a mystery. It does not occur in animals and so can only be studied in humans. It refers to those pregnancies that develop out of the womb, and while these have been reported in almost all sites in the upper genital tract the commonest site is the Fallopian tube. The pregnancies usually end early and this is accompanied by internal bleeding. The bleeding is generally heavy enough to need an emergency operation and can, very rarely, be enough to cause death. Most gynaecologists remove the damaged tube during the repair operation, which can have a catastrophic effect on the patient's future fertility.

Nobody really knows the reason for this apparent link between progestogen-only pill failures and ectopic pregnancies. Several suggestions have been made. The first, rather unlikely, explanation was the 'give-a-dog-a-bad-name-and-hang-it' theory. Some people felt that during the first few years that the progestogen-only pills were in use there were a few more than expected ectopic pregnancies. The new pills were then suspected and more damning evidence was sought. Every time there was another disaster the link became more firmly established in the minds of those who were unhappy with the new pills. Whenever a pill failure did not result in an ectopic pregnancy the fact was glossed over. Similarly, if someone using a different method of contraception had an ectopic pregnancy there was subconscious denial of the fact and the link between progestogen-only pills and ectopic pregnancy became established in folk-lore. A much more likely explanation, but one which is also impossible to prove, is that there is no real increase in the likelihood of ectopic pregnancy occurring when these pills fail. Progestogen-only pills work by making the womb inhospitable to the fertilized egg, but they do not necessarily stop the egg being fertilized. Thus, if the egg was one that was going to form an ectopic pregnancy by not passing along to the womb, there is nothing in the way this pill works to stop it doing this. The combined pills, on the other hand, will not only make conception less likely, they seem to act more strongly all the way along the genital tract. This suggests that the incidence of ectopic pregnancies in people taking progestogen-only pills is the same as for people who are not using any contraception. It is the combined pill which has a lower than normal rate of ectopic pregnancies. Similar arguments have been put forward about the links between the IUCD and ectopic pregnancy.

Another suggested explanation is that the effect of the progestogens leads to ectopic pregnancies. We have already mentioned that progestogens damp down the movements of the Fallopian tube, and they might slow it down so much that any fertilized egg in the tube would be unable to reach the womb. It would then remain in the tube and could possibly form an ectopic pregnancy. This is by no means certain. When fertilized eggs are deliberately put into the tubes, rather than the womb, of monkeys, ectopic pregnancies do not occur. This might be because of differences in the eggs or because something specific in the tubes of humans makes tubal implantation more likely. It has been suggested that the local action of progesterone is one of these factors, with damage caused by surgery or infection being other possible causes. It has also been suggested that this action of progesterone was one of the factors in the discovery that progesterone-loaded IUCDs had a relatively high rate of ectopic pregnancy when they failed. (This was higher than could have been expected for IUCDs in general.)

We should emphasize though that ectopic pregnancy is an extremely rare complication of using the progestogen-only pill. Neither of the authors has ever seen this happen despite the fact that we have both been working in the fields of gynaecological surgery and human reproduction for many years.

Reasons for using the progestogen-only pill

Many women are unsuitable for oestrogen-containing pills. They often benefit from, and are happy with, the progestogen-only pill. There are five main conditions in this category.

Contraception: the facts

Thrombosis

Progestogens do not increase the danger of blood-clotting. This has been confirmed by many laboratory studies that have looked carefully at all of the blood-clotting factors and have found minor changes in only one of them. Clinical studies have also shown that women treated with progestogens, even in high doses, do not have any increased risk of thrombosis, so that women who are at risk can use progestogen-only pills for contraception. These women include those who have had blood clots in their arteries or veins while previously taking oral contraceptives, or even out of the blue. Pulmonary embolus (i.e. blood clots in the blood-vessels of the lung) is the worst possible complication of these blood clots and women who have had one previously are advised to take progestogen-only pills. Unfortunately, the leaflets that drug companies give out with packets of their pills disagree with us. They are wrong because they have to be over-cautious. If you are worried about this, talk it over with your own doctor or a specialist adviser—see the last chapter for advice on this. Smokers are prone to developing disease of the blood-vessels, especially of those round the heart. It is important to make sure that the contraceptive method they use does not harm their health any more than their cigarettes do. Progestogen-only pills provide one such solution.

Being over 35

Progestogen-only pills also provide a solution to the contraceptive problems of the over 35 age group. One of the quirks of epidemiological research is that, of necessity, the people studied have to be put into neat little compartments which are not usually homogenous. For example, to make the study of age effects and the pill easier most epidemiologists divide women up into five-year age bands—30–34, 35–39, and so on. As women age they are more likely to develop heart and blood-vessel disease. This is a gradual process, with 45-year-old women being at a much greater risk than those who are 25. However, when survey data was analysed this process showed as a marked difference in the complication rates for those over, and those under, the age of 35. Some people who had not read the evidence came to the unfortunate conclusion that at the age of 35 women began to crumble and were unsuited to oral contraception. The ageing process is a gradual one, spread over decades, not starting at a definite time. Some 32-year-old women— those who smoke, are overweight, and have raised blood pressure—are unsuited to the pill already, while women who are 39, but slim, with normal blood pressure, and no heart and blood-vessel disease in their families are still suited to pills containing oestrogen. Nevertheless, many women approaching their 35th birthday do decide to change their contraceptive method. If they have been using the combined pill, the progestogen-only pill is often ideal for them. The failure rate we quoted earlier of one or two per 100 woman-years does not apply to them (since they are anyway less fertile at this age); it is probably much nearer to, or lower than, one unplanned pregnancy in every 200 woman-years of use.

High blood pressure

High blood pressure is another medical problem making some women unsuitable for oestrogen-containing pills. All oestrogen-containing pills raise blood pressure and, in the presence of raised blood pressure, diseases of the blood-vessels begin to occur. Progestogen-only pills are suitable for these women.

Breast-feeding

We mentioned in the last chapter that women who breast-feed may have a decrease in milk production when taking oestrogen-containing tablets. We shall discuss the effectiveness of breast-feeding as a contraceptive in Chapter 9, but

47

for many women this protection from pregnancy is not enough. They want added reassurance and this can be provided by the progestogen-only pill. It has almost no effect on milk production and almost none of the drug is passed into the milk.

Reasons for not using the progestogen-only pill

Not everyone is suited to these pills. The two main groups who would be ill-advised to take them are those with very heavy, frequent, and irregular periods, and those who have had an ectopic pregnancy. In addition, these pills are not suitable for young women who are desperately keen not to become pregnant. Women who have heavy, frequent, or irregular periods are not suited because their problem tends to get worse; women who have had an ectopic pregnancy are not suited because not only are they more likely to have a second ectopic pregnancy than someone who has never had one, but the treatment of a second such pregnancy is likely to leave them sterile. Many doctors will treat women with heavy or irregular periods with oral progestogens, but rather than using the progestogen-only pill they will use the same drug in much higher doses, using preparations like Primolut-N or Utovlan. These increased doses are of course still contraceptive.

Summary

Progestogen-only contraceptives are not widely used or known. Perhaps they deserve better publicity and there are encouraging signs that they are beginning to get it. They are widely used by women who have medical or social reasons for not using the combined pill. One of the problems that they pose is the fact that they need to be taken with great regularity and this is not always easy. A possible solution is the long-acting progestogens, which are discussed in the next chapter.

5

Long-acting progestogen contraception

In the previous two chapters we have discussed oral
contraception. Oral contraceptives are suitable for most
women, and their ease of use and effectiveness have made
them the most widely used form of medical contraception in
the world today. But, as we have discussed, they are not the
method of choice for all women. Oestrogens have side-
effects; the progesterone-only pill can cause a lot of irregular
bleeding; and the inconvenience of a daily tablet is more
than some women can put up with. For some of these
women—a small proportion in the United Kingdom but an
estimated one-and-a-half million world-wide—the solution
is a long-acting progestogen.

Experimental methods

Long-acting oral progestogens have never really lived up to
the hopes of expectations of scientists, and so the field
consists of only two varieties of long-acting injections and a
few experimental methods. We shall deal with the experimental methods first. They have all been tried out in
other parts of the world, principally Sweden, where they are
in limited use. None of these methods are as yet widely used
there, but all seem to have some promise. They consist of
silicone–plastic (silastic) cylinders that can be buried under
the skin, or vaginal rings, or hormone preparations wrapped
up in dissolvable wrappings. The small silastic cylinders leak
hormone gradually for several months. They have the
disadvantage that a small surgical operation is needed to
bury them under the skin. While this can be done as an
out-patient procedure, it still involves some discomfort, but
at least if the woman does not like the device it can easily be

removed. In theory, it can remain active for five to seven years.

Silastic vaginal rings were developed a few years ago. They are hollow rings, resembling a thin plastic doughnut. They have a hormone-filled core which leaks hormone continuously. There is usually enough hormone to last for six months or so, and this steady leakage of hormone is enough to suppress ovulation, production of cervical mucus, and very often menstruation for all that time. When the woman wants a pregnancy, or a period, or the six months are up, she removes the device herself and fits a new one.

Hormone preparations wrapped in coatings that can be broken down inside the body are an exciting new idea. They consist of tiny spheres of either pure progesterone or a progestogen surrounded by a skin which is made of a synthetic polymer that is destroyed by the body to give simple, non-harmful by-products like lactic acid or glucose. The size of the sphere determines the rate at which it is broken down, and so the rate at which the hormone inside is released. The whole preparation is a collection of millions of tiny spheres, all designed to dissolve over a period of several months. Some disintegrate on the first day and just as many on the two-hundredth. Since all of the ingredients are either natural body hormones or tried and tested polymers that break down to simple compounds which are easily handled by the body, it is possible that, after more clinical trials, these preparations might be available for use soon.

Types of long-acting progestogen

Most of these methods are still in the future. For most women the choice in long-acting progestogens is between two long-acting injections—depot micro-crystalline med-roxy-progesterone acetate (Depo-Provera), and norethisterone oenanthate (Noristerat). These are very different drugs but with a similar aim—to provide a high circulating level of progestogen, which will switch off ovulation, and to have a direct effect on the endometrium and cervical mucus. Both have the same disadvantage. In the first few days after an injection the levels of the drug in the bloodstream are often high enough to give side-effects. This level then settles to an acceptable one for several weeks, followed by the complete removal of the drug from the body and a return to normality.

Depo-Provera

Depo-Provera consists of micro-crystals of different sizes, containing the drug. It is the older of the two preparations and has been in clinical use for over 20 years, which is long enough for its benefits and problems to have been identified. It was first used in the treatment of uterine cancer, where it is still one of the hormone treatments used. It was then tried as an agent to treat pregnant women who were going into premature labour. While its use in the treatment of uterine cancer is well-established, its use in treating premature labour has been abandoned—but then, nothing else seems to work either! It was noticed that women who received large doses—up to 30 times the dosages now in use—had many months with no periods after childbirth. This led to its being tried as a contraceptive, and the first published work appeared in 1963 based on two years' experience.

Noristerat

Norethisterone oenanthate (Noristerat) is a newer preparation and was first tried in 1966. Unlike Depo-Provera it depends for its action on the slow release of active hormone from the oily base in which it is injected, and then slow breakdown by enzymes in the body to give pure norethisterone. Norethisterone was one of the first progestogens to be synthesized and it is still one of the main ones used in oral contraception, both alone and in combination with oestrogens. This preparation is less long-lasting than Depo-

Provera, with most of the normal dose being removed from the body in about 60 days.

How these drugs act

Both Depo-Provera and Noristerat act in a similar fashion and are broadly similar to the progestogen-only pill that we discussed in the previous chapter. The main difference is that these preparations have a much more profound effect on ovulation than the pills—they stop ovulation altogether in a great many cases. This contributes to an effect on the endometrium, the cervical mucus, and the Fallopian tube.

Side-effects

The fact that these injections stop ovulation means that they stop periods and this, coupled with the fact that they make the lining of the womb less active, causes irregular episodes of bleeding. Women tend to have lighter, scantier periods with more bleeding in between periods, but this is not always the case. Some women do not bleed at all while, very rarely, some women get heavy, continuous episodes of bleeding, sometimes necessitating treatment in hospital. As treatment with these drugs continues the women tend to have fewer and lighter periods, with many eventually having none at all. This is more of a problem with Depo-Provera than with Noristerat. Although many women are delighted to have lighter periods, most of the women who stop using the drug give this as the main reason for doing so.

How the drugs are administered

These drugs are injected into the buttocks every three months (for Depo-Provera) or two to three months (for Noristerat). The exact timing of injections for Noristerat is still being debated. When the injections were given every three months about 3 per cent of the women got pregnant every year. Most doctors now suggest that they are given every eight weeks for the first six months and then every three months. Both drugs are rather thick, oily solutions, Noristerat more so than Depo-Provera. Most clinics warm Noristerat before giving it, since that makes it less treacle-like and a less painful injection. The injections are usually given within the first few days of the start of a period, which provides protection from then on and makes sure that these long-acting compounds are not inadvertently given to someone who might be pregnant. Depo-Provera was used for the treatment of premature labour, and to try and treat those women who were beginning to miscarry, and had no obvious ill-effects on the babies from those pregnancies, so it is probably perfectly safe to give to pregnant women.

Advantages

Both drugs have many good points in their favour. It is ironic that the features that make them suitable for some women are also those that have made them unpopular with others. They are obviously much easier to administer than daily tablets and are much less prone to 'patient error'. Once they have been given the drugs remain active for 8 to 12 weeks, and during that period their effect cannot be reversed by antibiotics or anti-epileptic drugs. (This means of course that women who decide they do not like them are unable to do much about it except wait for them to be cleared from the body.)

The fact that they do not increase the danger of blood-clotting, and almost certainly lack an effect on the inner walls of blood-vessels, makes them ideal for those women who have had a blood-vessel thrombosis in the past. Neither do they seem to affect blood pressure or the way in which the body handles glucose. This makes them suitable for women with high blood pressure or diabetes.

Disadvantages

The preparations are associated with some problems though. The biggest single one is their effect on menstrual bleeding. Almost invariably women who have been taking these preparations for a long time get long episodes—sometimes several months at a time—without bleeding. This can be worrying because most sexually active women associate this with pregnancy, but after this has been explained to them the next main concern they have is of permanent, unintentional infertility. There is in fact no evidence that infertility is caused, but, because sexuality and fertility are very closely interlinked in our culture, the thought of potential infertility is worrying for women. There are no other significant complications of their use.

The biggest worry that has been put forward about these drugs is their link with cancer. In some of the early experiments with beagle bitches who were given extremely large doses, some of them developed breast nodules. Dogs break-down drugs like Depo-Provera in a completely different way from humans and nowadays it has been realized that beagle bitches are particularly unsuited to drug trials of this sort. They have a very high rate of spontaneous development of breast nodules and in the United Kingdom the Committee on the Safety of Medicines, which is the government watch-dog on all drugs, has now recommended that in future no tests be carried out using these animals.

When other trials were carried out on very small numbers of monkeys, who were given 50 times the normal dose of Depo-Provera for several years, two developed uterine cancer. Again the significance is unclear. Monkeys do not have the same sort of womb and womb lining that humans do and studies on small numbers who were given inordinately large doses of the drug probably have no direct relevance to humans. Most drug safety bodies in Western Europe, including the United Kingdom Committee on the Safety of

Long-acting progestogen contraception

Medicines, have now approved the drug for clinical use. This accords with the clinical viewpoint, that studies in many countries have shown no change in patterns of cancer in women, and we would expect long-term use to be associated with reductions in uterine and ovarian cancer for the same reasons that progestogen-containing oral contraceptives are.

Reasons for using long-acting progestogens

These preparations have two main uses as contraceptives. They can be used in all circumstances where oral progestogens are suitable, and they also fulfil a role—sometimes a very controversial one—in the care of women who are unable to use oral progestogens. Sometimes this can be for medical reasons. This group includes those women who have had major bowel surgery, in which a large part of the bowel has been removed, or have some other form of bowel disease that prevents them from effectively absorbing tablets. Much more commonly, women are unable to take tablets for social reasons and either the doctor decides the woman is unable to take tablets regularly or the woman herself makes this decision. Occasionally a woman finds that her home environment is unsuitable for easy contraception. This might be because her partner objects to all forms of contraception or because her life-style is too erratic to permit regular contraceptive use. For example, one of the authors was once consulted by an airline stewardess who was terrified of becoming pregnant, but was also very worried that her frequent trips around the world, with constant time-changes, led to very large gaps in her pill-taking; a once-in-three-months injection was ideal for her.

The biggest problem comes with those women whom their doctor feels will be unable to take oral contraception daily or use a method like the diaphragm effectively. The problem is very often one of the doctor's attitudes rather than the woman's motivation. Many of these women tend to be of lower than average intelligence, higher than average fertility, and are very often unmarried and unemployed. The use of any form of contraception over which these women have no direct control is controversial. It has eugenic overtones and if, as sometimes happens, the women are black, and the doctors white, then racial elements creep into the dispute.

In a London hospital recently three-quarters of all women who went home after having their babies did so after receiving an injection of one of these drugs. In many cases they had had no discussion about the reasons for this and some were not even aware of having received a contraceptive injection. They certainly did not give informed consent. It is instances like this that have led to fears of compulsory medication and have fuelled so much of the debate over the issue.

In the United Kingdom, unlike most other countries (including most of Western Europe), only one form of contraceptive injection has been licensed, and this initially only for limited use. This preparation (Depo-Provera) was licensed in Britain for the use of women who are waiting the results of their husband's vasectomy (see Chapter 10) or who are trying to avoid pregnancy while waiting for German measles vaccine to work. Both of these are regarded as short-term uses and the last is probably unnecessary—there is no evidence that rubella vaccine given before or during pregnancy is harmful to the baby. Most doctors who are involved in family planning work disagree with this point of view and use Depo-Provera for a much bigger population of woman, and since the successful legal appeal in 1984 they have been able to do so openly.

In the United States of America the Food and Drug Administration is currently holding an enquiry into the safety of Depo-Provera and the results of this are expected to make Depo-Provera more widely available.

It is unfortunate that most of the problems of heavy, extra bleeding occur in the first three months of use, and so the link between Depo-Provera and bleeding problems is being strengthened by the large numbers of women who use it for short periods of time only.

The future

The future does not look bright for this form of contraception. It is safe, it is effective, and there is a demand for it from women and their health workers. But it has a bad image, which makes workers within the field of contraception chary of pressing for its wider use, and women themselves worried about the social consequences of its widespread use. The situation may improve in the future.

6

Barrier methods of contraception

> Rubbers are jolly,
> Rubbers are fun.
> Better to use one,
> Than end up a mum!

This was the winning entry in a recent American competition, aimed at schoolchildren, to find a simple jingle that would help to popularize the condom. It is typical of the recent changes in public attitudes to the use of barrier contraceptives. For many decades they were the only available means of effective contraception, but with the advent of the oral contraceptive pill their use declined. Now their popularity is increasing, and with this (or maybe because of this) there has been a change in public attitudes.

History

The condom

Barrier methods have a long history. The earliest recorded barriers were used by the ancient Egyptians and consisted of honey-coated pessaries. The original reason for using the honey-coating was probably sexual, but the realization that it prevented pregnancy must have been responsible for its continued use; honey is effective at killing both spermatozoa and bacteria. The men of ancient Egypt also used a form of barrier contraception; some of the tomb paintings show men wearing penile coverings of brightly coloured linen. Again, the initial reason may have been sexual attractiveness, followed by the realization that there was a contraceptive effect.

In the eighteenth century Casanova recommended the use

of half-lemons as a vaginal barrier contraceptive. Like the earlier honey-coated pessaries this had a dual action with the lemon acting as a physical barrier to sperms and the acid in it killing any stray sperms. In his youth Casanova was extremely vociferous in his condemnation of the early contraceptive sheaths and was quoted as saying 'do not wait to see me close myself up in a piece of dead skin . . . to prove to you that I am perfectly alive'. People like him are responsible for the centuries-old association between the sheath and illicit sex or venereal disease. A hundred years before him Mme de Sévigné held similar views—she described condoms to her daughter as being 'armour against love, gossamer against infection'. Some authorities believe that the condom is named after Dr Condom, the physician to King Charles II who recommended that the King use sheaths made of either oiled linen or the intestines of sheep. These were to prevent the birth of illegitimate children and protect the King from venereal disease.

Casanova began to appreciate the advantages of the condom after catching venereal disease, and when he was in his mid-thirties said: 'Ten months ago I would have called this [the condom] an invention of the devil, but now I find that its inventor must have been a man of goodwill.' Many men had their first contact with 'rubber prophylactics' when they were issued with them in the Armed Forces. The idea that condoms were, and for many people still are, associated with disease and illicit sex, was reinforced by the practice of issuing them in the Forces to prevent servicemen from getting venereal disease. Marie Stopes had a different reason for disapproving of condoms. In her 1923 book *Contraception* she wrote that 'women absorb from the seminal fluid of the man some substance, "hormone", "vitamine" or stimulant which affects their internal economy in such a way as to benefit and nourish their whole system'. She approved of the sheath for use only on the wedding night, because she felt that newly married women might be so upset at the sight or feel of recently ejaculated semen that it could have profound effects on the relationship.

The diaphragm

An interesting link between public attitudes to sex and barrier contraception emerged with attempts to publicize the diaphragm for women. In many parts of the world local laws on obscenity prevented the sale or importation of contraceptive diaphragms, and many doctors had qualms about being associated with them. Dr C. Hasse, who was one of the early workers in the field, used the pseudonym Wilhelm P.J. Mensinga to protect his reputation. It is interesting to note that in his article '*Ueber facultative Sterilität*' ('On facultative sterility', his term for planned sterility, or contraception) he did not once mention the diaphragm by name, and his list of uses for contraception was remarkable for its shortness, including only 'good medical' reasons for avoiding childbirth. Dr Margaret Sanger tried to take some diaphragms back to the USA in the early part of this century but the Comstock laws, banning the importation of pornography and contraceptives, prevented this. She was forced to wait for many years until an American company began manufacturing the diaphragm there.

The argument has been made that the diaphragm is a sexually liberating device for women. It was the first reliable contraceptive device over which they had control and to use it they needed to be able to examine themselves and understand their own sexual anatomy. This is said to instil a greater confidence in their own abilities to control their fertility. Even in the last quarter of the twentieth century there are still many women who do not have a clear idea about the anatomy and physiology of their reproductive organs. It was the explicit nature of the necessary instruction that made the early pioneers fall foul of the obscenity laws, laws that had been passed during Victorian times.

Barrier methods of contraception

Types of barrier contraception

This chapter will consider three main types of barrier contraception. We will first discuss the sheath, or condom, which is the only effective form of reversible male contraception that is currently available. The female barriers, of which the diaphragm, or Dutch cap, is the most important, will be considered next and, finally, the spermicidal preparations. Most authorities say that spermicides should not be used on their own but in conjunction with other barrier methods. We will consider the various types of foams, gels, and creams in the last part of the chapter. Natural barriers will be dealt with in Chapter 9, while in Chapter 12 we shall discuss the future in contraception, which includes several new forms of barrier contraception for women.

The condom

Modern production of condoms began with the development of the rubber industry in the second half of the last century. The manufacturing technique is relatively simple; cylindrical moulds are dipped into tanks of latex and the sheath is then rolled off. Nearly all sheaths are now made in bulk by big machines but there are a few factories, principally in the Third World, where they are still made by hand.

The most important part of condom manufacture comes after they are made. Quality control is important but still depends on not necessarily relevant tests. Most manufacturers test a few condoms from each batch by filling them with water, usually 300 ml, or sometimes 25 litres of air. The idea behind this is that if the sheath bursts with a large volume of air or water it is likely to be substandard, and probably so are many others in the batch. Some makers also roll the water-filled sheath on blotting paper and count it as a failure if there is any staining of the paper. Some manufacturers routinely do a more scientific test on all condoms they produce by measuring the electrical conductivity of the rubber. A well-formed, intact, rubber sheath should be a good insulator of electricity. The condoms are put into a bath of salty water and an electric current is passed from an electrode inside the sheath. Ideally the condom should insulate the electrode inside the sheath from the one outside in the water bath, and any leakage of electricity implies a hole in the sheath through which the salty water can leak. The Japanese standard, for instance, demands a resistance of at least 200 000 ohms.

Another test is to cut a small square of rubber from the side of a sample and stretch it on a machine to see how much force is needed to tear it. This test is claimed to be more rigorous, but the argument has been put forward that the results are not directly relevant to condom use—but then neither is putting in 300 ml of water! In the early days of condom manufacture, dust particles and similar imperfections led to flaws in the latex sheets causing tears. Nowadays this is less likely since most factories are isolated from the outside environment.

There is still argument about the importance of holes in condoms. A broken sheath is obviously of no use as a barrier, but microscopic holes, detectable only with delicate machines, are unlikely to let sufficient sperms through to be a hazard. However, there is concern that they might let bacteria through. (Remember that one of the earliest permitted uses for the condom was as a prophylactic against venereal disease.)

How to use the condom. Many people who read this book will at some stage of their lives have had some experience of condoms. Even so, it is worth re-emphasizing some of the rules for using them safely and effectively. Figure 3 shows a condom in place.

One of the important rules in safe condom use is to use them together with spermicides. The spermicides 'mop-up' sperms that might leak out from the base of the condom and

Barrier methods of contraception

are an additional protection should the (uncommon) disaster of sheath breakage occur.

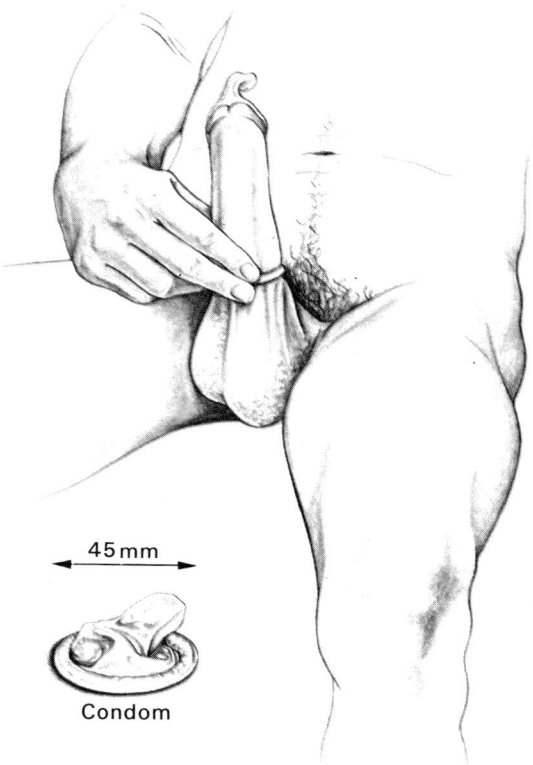

45 mm

Condom

Fig 3. Putting on a condom.

Some of the fluid produced from the tip of the penis when men become aroused contains spermatozoa, and so it is important to put the condom on at the start of sexual activity. Since it is very difficult to put a condom on a soft penis, this means that couples must break off from foreplay to put the condom on as soon as the erection is hard enough. This must be before any vaginal contact by the penis. Many

63

men find this the hardest thing of all to do because they feel that attention is being focused on their penis at a most crucial time. For some men, this is part of sexual foreplay and they enjoy it. For others, it is embarrassing and causes feelings of inadequacy.

Once ejaculation has occurred the penis should be withdrawn and the condom removed. There should be no more close genital contact because, even though most condoms are covered with spermicides, there may still be some living sperms on the outside of the penis. Some couples find this the hardest part to accept in using the condom—to them close personal contact after intercourse is deeply satisfying and they resent having to separate at this time.

What to do if the condom breaks. If the condom does break, or come off, then post-coital contraception should be used. This is discussed in Chapter 8, and one of the advantages of its widespread availability is that couples using the sheath can do so with the knowledge that should an accident occur the worst consequences can be avoided.

Nobody is sure of the mechanisms of sheath breakage. There are several important factors, both in the design and the use of the device. One of the most controversial features in the design of the sheath is its thickness. In his book *The politics of contraception* Carl Djerassi emphasizes this point, and that the official regulations in the USA produce the thickest condoms in the world. The shortest permissible American condom is one centimetre longer than the longest permitted Hungarian condom! Djerassi feels that if American condoms were thinner they would be more widely accepted. However, in some societies, where there are no governmental restrictions and the markets are more openly competitive than in the West, there is no evidence that consumer pressure is producing a market for thinner condoms. This is particularly true of Singapore. Some companies do emphasize the thinness of their products to try and boost sales, but there is little evidence that this is an important factor in consumer choice.

Another problem in the use of the condom is its packaging. Some people are concerned that the sharp edges of the foil packs may tear the condom, while the transparent plastic of other packets may expose it to light and let the rubber deteriorate. Since many coloured condoms are sold in packets that are transparent on one side and foil on the other it could be argued that these are getting the worst of both worlds! In addition, not much is known about the effect of ageing on condoms. There is probably no reason to think that the rubber will perish in anything less than several years, and there are few couples who keep them that long. Perhaps inefficient family planning bureaucracies in some Third World countries allow this to happen, but this is unlikely. Schoolboys are notorious for carrying the same condom around in their pockets for months on end without ever using it. It is a badge of manhood for them, but the damage that can be done when it is treated like this makes it a pretty risky one!

The last feature we will discuss in condom design is probably the most controversial one. The American sex researchers Masters and Johnson established that under laboratory conditions most penises are the same size when erect. Condoms used to be manufactured in one standard size but this is not the case nowadays. In 1972 the United States Agency for International Development sent standard Western condoms to Bangladesh. With amusement these were rejected and they are now supplied two centimetres shorter and three millimetres smaller in diameter. The American writer Barbara Seaman, when testifying before Congress in Washington, suggested that since women bought brassieres with differing cup sizes, so men should buy condoms in differing sizes. To protect male egos she suggested that they be labelled jumbo, colossal, and supercolossal! Neither she nor anyone else has published any evidence that poorly fitting condoms are more likely to burst, or leak around the edges, than well fitting ones. Since condoms are fairly strong, and rubber does stretch, most authorities are unconvinced by these arguments.

Apart from the errors in use that we mentioned earlier, there are two other aspects of condom use that make accidents likely. Again, it is very difficult to know how common each of these particular problems is. The first occurs when the condom is being rolled on. If either partner has sharp finger-nails then the condom can be torn. The jagged edges of bitten nails are said to be worse for this than elegantly manicured ones. Small tears and nicks can go unnoticed but could be the starting-point for much larger ones.

Vaginal dryness can also lead to damage. As women become sexually aroused the vaginal walls moisten and this lubrication helps intercourse. Similarly, men secrete fluid from the tip of the penis which also helps penetration. Most condoms are lubricated with silicone oil but, for some people, this is not moist enough and the condom can be torn. If vaginal dryness is a problem it can be treated with either a lubricant, like KY jelly, or a contraceptive jelly like Duragel. However, the problem might lie in over-hasty insertion of the penis, and more relaxed intercourse with more foreplay might be a better solution.

Modern rubber technology has meant that condoms can now be manufactured in a great variety of colours, shapes and textures. There is no evidence that women find textured condoms more satisfying than the traditional ones, but the important thing about these changes is that they make more people aware of condoms, and prepared to discuss them, and, it is hoped, use them. It has been recognized for millennia that colours can be used to heighten sexual attractiveness and this has lead to the recent interest in colouring condoms. An interesting point about this is that in Sweden one of the most popular condom colours is black, while in Kenya it is white!

Although it is widely used the condom is often not the first choice of contraception for many couples. It has been suggested that it is very useful for couples who have intercourse infrequently, where it is often a most acceptable method, especially where backed up by morning-after contraception for the occasional failures. It has also been recommended for young people since it avoids the potentially embarrassing visits to a clinic that can disturb them, while at the same time providing some protection against infection. Most authorities would say that for them a better method of contraception is probably the pill.

Reliability. It is not possible to quote failure rates for condoms. Most textbooks say that for every hundred couples who use sheaths for a year, between one and five will have an unwanted pregnancy. This ignores the fact that many of the couples who use condoms are doing so between contraceptive methods, and are only using the condom for a short period of time. Also, many of the original surveys did not count on women being able to get post-coital contraception if there was an accident with the sheath. In most parts of the world most couples who use the condom do so without contacting doctors and family planning clinics, and this means that statistics on the regularity of use, and the use of spermicides as well, are hard to come by. The couples who are seen in family planning clinics asking for a change of method are probably an atypical, biased sample. Several studies have shown that couples who were determined not to have another pregnancy have had failure rates of less than one for every hundred couples using them for a year.

The diaphragm

Most people accept that the diaphragm is a more efficient barrier (from the point of view of stopping pregnancy) than the condom, though no-one knows why! Figure 4 shows two diaphragms of different sizes. For many years these were the only available effective form of female contraception and fitting them was almost an art form. People were so certain that accurate fitting was essential that the caps came in sizes only 2½ mm apart. Some pioneer teachers would demonstrate on themselves the correct way to fit a cap up to twenty times a day. It could even be that it was this sort of activity that offended some of the legal authorities who banned the importation of female contraceptives into the USA for so many years. Recently attitudes have begun to change. Some of these changes were introduced after researchers studied the way that the body changed during sexual activity. Two decades ago Masters and Johnson found that during sexual excitement the upper two-thirds of the vagina expands outwards, increasing in volume. This ballooning means that something that was a good fit at a clinic would be poorly fitting right at the moment it was needed. The fact that the rim is made of a steel spring helps to keep the fit better than it might be otherwise but still does not compensate for all the changes that can occur.

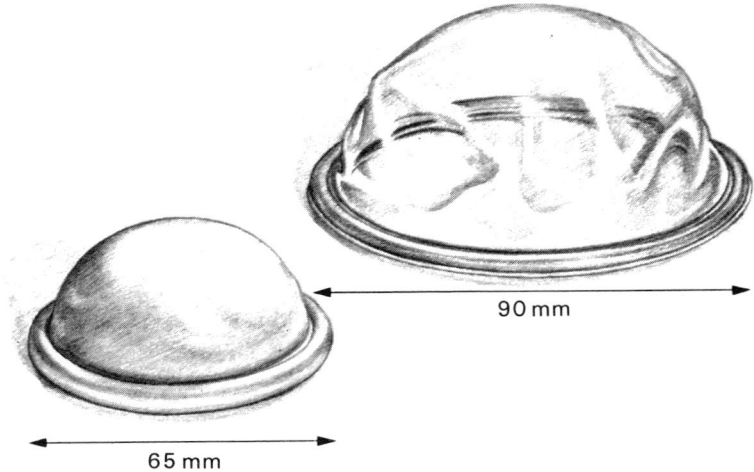

90 mm

65 mm

Fig. 4. The diaphragm.

Barrier methods of contraception

In 1980 a New York gynaecologist began to dispense with another of the hallowed traditions. Rather than fit women with the largest size diaphragm they could comfortably wear, he began to advocate that all women should be fitted with the same sized small one. The results of this were promising but, before abandoning the time-honoured methods, we need to evaluate this new technique properly.

For decades it was taught that one of the functions of the diaphragm was to provide a relatively immobile platform for holding spermicidal cream against the cervix. The idea was that any sperms that got past the rubber would be eliminated by the cream, and it was this twofold mechanism of action that was considered so important. However, nobody has ever proved this, and the New York gynaecologist mentioned earlier has suggested that perhaps small caps with no spermicide are as effective as larger ones with cream.

One of the advantages of the recent upsurge of interest in barrier contraception is that perhaps some of these questions are going to be answered now. Several centres have begun scientifically conducted trials comparing differing types of these devices, and perhaps the second edition of this book will have more information. There is an immense lack of knowledge and this has even led to some legal problems. One form of vaginal barrier that we shall discuss later is the cervical cap. This little-used device is made only in the United Kingdom, and the United States Food and Drug Administration (the FDA), which is their watchdog over all forms of medicines, has labelled this a 'significant risk device'. Their point of view is simple—until 1982 there had been no published research on the cervical cap since 1953, during which time our attitudes to drug safety and contraception have undergone significant changes. The upshot of this is that since July 1980 the only people who can supply the cap are those who are conducting research into it and have registered their research programme with the FDA. Until there is more, and new, evidence on its safety and effectiveness they do not want to expose American women to what they consider might be a hazardous device.

How to use the diaphragm.   Using the vaginal diaphragm is simple but needs practice. As with any device that needs skill, the only people drawn to it are those who are motivated and prepared to persevere. This means that many of the couples who do use these methods are highly motivated and, as we discussed in Chapter 13, the evidence is that for all forms of contraception these people have better success rates. It has also been suggested, rather unkindly, that the amount of fiddling needed and the degree of perseverance required means that only those with low sex drives are likely to continue using the cap for a long period of time.

The first essential point in using the cap is to have it in place before it is needed. Most women who use it will put it in every time that they are likely to have sex, recognizing that they will only use it on some of those occasions. Most authorities still say that the cap should be used along with spermicidal cream and so this needs to be smeared on to the cap first. Most of the creams and jellies are also lubricants and these help with the insertion of what can be a rather springy device. The side that is going to be up against the cervix needs to have most of the cream.

There are many ways of fitting the device. For any woman the best way is the one she finds most comfortable, and this can only be found out by her, or her and her partner, experimenting in comfort and privacy. Most women find that one of the easiest approaches is to put one foot on a raised surface, for instance the edge of a bath or lavatory, and pass the cap upwards and backwards. Other women prefer to squat or lie on their backs. As a form of foreplay some women let their partners insert the device, which also helps the men to assume some of the responsibility for contraception. The device is squeezed lengthways along its mid-portion and then pushed upwards and backwards, rather like a tampon would be. It is then checked to make sure that it is covering the cervix and is comfortably nestled against the pubic bone. Once the device is in it must be left in place for at least six hours after intercourse. If sex occurs more than once in that period then more spermicides will be needed. Since the cap cannot be taken out to put more on, a syringe-like applicator, to squirt more cream into the vagina, or pessary pushed up to the top of the vagina will be required.

When the cap is taken out it must be cleaned, dried, and replaced in its container. Most caps will last for a couple of years but it is a good idea to change them after this time. A skilled person should check that they are being worn correctly several times a year, and sooner after a pregnancy or if there is a change of several pounds in body-weight. A weight change of about ten pounds or more may affect the size and shape of the vagina and thus the fit of the cap.

Types of diaphragm.   Not every woman is suited to the diaphragm, although the wide range of diaphragms available do suit most women. There are four main types of diaphragm and if they are not suitable then there are three other types of vaginal barriers—the cervical cap, the vault cap, and the vimule. We will discuss some of the newer types of barrier in Chapter 12 on recent advances and future prospects in contraception.

We shall first discuss the two most widely used of the four types of diaphragm. The *coil spring* type has a spiral coiled steel spring in the rim. It is particularly suitable for women with strong vaginal muscles and a normally shaped and sized vagina, with a womb that leans forwards rather than backwards. The shelf behind the pubic bone (on which the device rests) must also be deep and firm.

The *Mensinga diaphragm*, a *flat spring* device, has a flat

71

band of springy steel in the rim. It is firmer than the coil spring diaphragm and is particularly suitable for women with a shallow arch behind the pubic bone. Many of the women who find this device comfortable have never had their birth passages stretched by having babies.

The *arcing spring* diaphragm has features of both the coil spring and the flat spring diaphragms. There is a double metal spring in the rim and this produces a lot of pressure. This makes the device ideal for those women with lax vaginal muscles and some degree of prolapse. Because of the extra pressure that the ring has on the pelvis, if the diaphragm is not fitted carefully it can cause pain and even lead to difficulty in passing urine.

The *Matrisalus diaphragm* is a fairly infrequently used version with a strong flat steel band in the rim. This is curved instead of being round, and this gives an added lift to the front wall of the vagina. It is useful in women who have laxity of the wall, but because of its odd shape it is more difficult to fit than the other three types.

There are many skills that cannot be learned from books and fitting diaphragms is one of them. Women who want to use this method of contraception should really go to a clinic where there is an expert who fits many of them. More than any other type of contraception this one is not for the occasional amateur to prescribe.

The last three types of female barrier contraceptive are those that are uncommonly used. They are the *cervical cap* (Fig. 5), the *vault cap* (Fig. 6), and the *vimule* (Fig. 7). They are all used by those women who are unable to use a diaphragm because of weak vaginal muscles. They sit high in the vagina and are held against the cervix by suction. They are much more difficult to apply and use of them has declined to almost negligible proportions over the past decade. Even the recent upsurge in interest has come too late to rescue manufacture of them, with only one company (in England) still making them.

Barrier methods of contraception

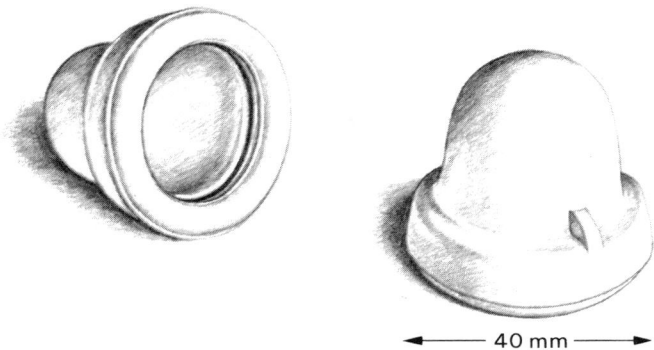

Fig. 5. The vimule.

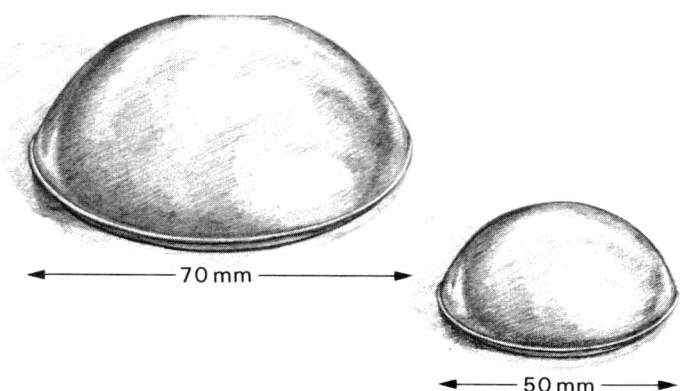

Fig. 6. The cervical cap.

Spermicides

The last, and in many ways the most important, form of barrier contraception are the spermicides. Physical barriers on their own are rarely sufficient and nearly all authorities recommend that they are backed up with chemical spermicides. If women use only spermicides there is a chance that between 10 and 20 in every 100 using them will get pregnant in each year of use, but the combination of spermicides and

73

Contraception: the facts

barriers, if used carefully, has a failure rate of less than five pregnancies per year for each 100 women using them. Spermicides are little used now and their relatively high failure rate is one of the reasons for this. The other major reason is that they are, or have the reputation of being, very 'messy'. They are much more widely available now than they were in 1881 when Charles Bradlaugh and Annie Besant went on trial for reprinting a pamphlet that advocated douching with weak solutions of chemicals after intercourse. The publicity that their trial caused took sales of the pamphlet from 1000 copies a year to 185 000 in the next 40 months. Douching is not a very effective method of contraception as explained on p.95.

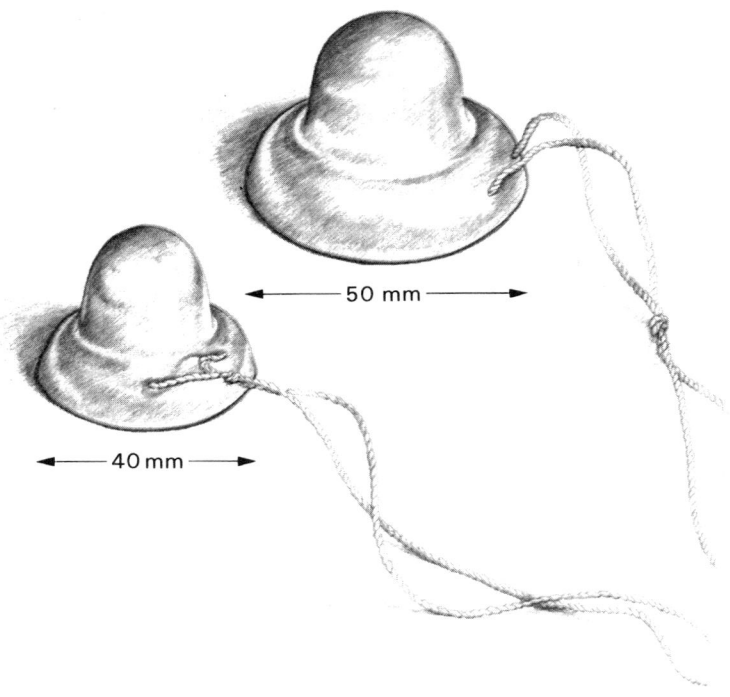

50 mm

40 mm

Fig. 7. The vault cap.

Barrier methods of contraception

There are six main types of spermicidal preparation available nowadays. All have the same basic aim—to deliver high concentrations of spermicidal drugs to the area around the neck of the womb in order to kill as many sperms as possible before they swim into the mucus from the cervix. Because the sperm can swim into the safety of the mucus within a few seconds of ejaculation, spermicides must act rapidly and also have the ability to spread over the whole of the area around the cervix (since they are unlikely to have been put into exactly the right spot). The sperm-killing action is produced by the chemical agent in the spermicide. There used to be many of these chemicals, some of them quite powerful acids and others derived from mercury. Concern about the possible long-term health hazards has whittled the number down and only two chemicals are now being used. The commonest is nonoxynol-9 (the name of which is the shortened version of a 29-letter compound). This chemical attaches itself to the outer surface of spermatozoa and stops them from taking in oxygen. It also upsets the surface tension forces that hold the outer skin of sperms together. By itself it is fairly effective in the test-tube but ineffective on its own in real life. It needs to be carried to the place where it will do the most harm to the spermatozoa and that is the function of the carrier base. This base determines the spermicide's action and how it is used.

Pessaries. Pessaries, small tablets that are put into the vagina, have either a wax or a water-soluble base. They are sometimes known as suppositories, particularly in the USA. They have the advantage of being portable with one complete dose being wrapped up in foil or plastic. They need to be inserted high up in the vagina, ideally about 15 minutes before intercourse, so that they can melt and allow the sper-micide to spread over the whole area. One study carried out in the USA found that women were unhappy at using them, because they felt that having to anticipate intercourse by 15 minutes ruined the spontaneity of the event!

Creams.   Creams are based on oil or fat preparations. They tend not to spread far from where they are put and so need to be used with care. They can be smeared on to the outside of a diaphragm or a syringe-like applicator can be used to insert them high into the vagina.

Jellies.   Jellies are based on gelatin. This melts rapidly at body temperature and so spreads over the whole of the vagina easily. They can be used, like the creams, on the outside of diaphragms. A syringe-like applicator can be used to put jelly into the vagina. Both creams and jellies can be used in conjunction with condoms or an IUCD or when intercourse occurs more than once in six hours for women using diaphragms. In practice there is very little difference between creams and jellies and most women would be best advised to use the one they find suits them.

Foaming tablets.   Foaming tablets release lots of bubbles of carbon dioxide when they become wet. These bubbles spread the spermicide throughout the vagina and the small bubbles help to provide a network that traps the sperms. They are similar in action to the pessaries but probably more effective. An interesting new foaming tablet that is used widely throughout the world, but not yet in the United Kingdom, is Neo-Sampoon, which was developed about twenty years ago in Japan. The basis for the action is Menfegol, a newer spermicide. Two of the selling points for this preparation are that it is said to be more effective at killing sperms than older spermicidal preparations, and also that it provides a feeling of warmth as it foams. This was considered a side-effect at first, and upset women, but when the company changed their advertising policy to emphasize this, sales improved!

Foaming aerosols.   Foaming aerosols work on the same

principle as the tablets but the bubbles are formed by gas under high pressure in an aerosol container. Care should be taken when loading the syringe applicator otherwise foam can be sprayed all over the bedroom. One of the advantages that aerosols have over creams and jellies is that, because they use compressed gas, they take up little bulk and so a month's supply can easily be kept in a small handbag.

C-film. C-film is the only contraceptive that is said to be suitable for use by both men and women. It is a spermicide-impregnated film that can either be pushed up on to the cervix or worn on the tip of the penis. The idea is that the film will dissolve in a few minutes and spread nonoxynol-9 over either the penis or the cervix. The films are infrequently used now because of their unacceptably high failure rate.

Reliability. Spermicides should not be used on their own because, without the assistance of another method, they are not effective enough at stopping a pregnancy. They have been recommended as adjuncts to the IUCD to reduce its already low failure rate to still lower levels, but their main use is with the barriers. When carefully used together with the diaphragm or condom the joint effectiveness of the two approaches that of the pill. A few studies have suggested that with some spermicides and some groups of women the failure rate approaches that of unprotected intercourse! Most studies though put the failure rate at between 5 and 15 in every 100 women using them for a year.

Their ease and availability is simultaneously one of their strongest and weakest points. In general any method of contraception that can be easily obtained is to be welcomed, because one of the most important factors in contraception is getting people to use it. At the same time, perhaps the fact that spermicides are so widely available engenders in some women a false sense of security. Perhaps they should be freely available, but with a little warning note to say that on their own they are not sufficient and should really be used alongside another method.

Effects on pregnancy.   Why should we be concerned about pregnancies occurring when these preparations have failed? There are two main reasons. Perhaps the most important is that any unplanned pregnancy, even though it may not be unwanted, is always to be regretted. Pregnancies ideally should be entered into in a positive frame of mind, not accepted as an occasional complication of contraception.

Another important reason though is that there is increasing evidence of a link between the use of spermicides at the time of conception, or perhaps within the months before conception, and abnormalities in the babies that result. The evidence is still not conclusive and investigations are still going on, but there have been consistent similarities in results between several large studies carried out by different groups in several parts of the world, principally the USA. The risk is slight but measurable.

Summary.   Spermicides are an effective adjunct to other methods of contraception. On their own they are not effective enough but they do improve other methods. They are cheap and freely available. There are no significant side-effects from their use, apart from the provisos about pregnancy, with not only a greater likelihood of its occurring than with other methods of contraception, but also a possibly greater likelihood of an abnormal pregnancy developing. The disadvantages that couples find with them are usually purely personal—objections to their messiness or their taste.

7

The intrauterine contraceptive device (IUCD)

The intrauterine contraceptive device (IUCD) is what we commonly also know as 'the coil'. The name conjures up a nasty image to a lot of people, and many women whom we see are amazed to find what a small and simple device the modern coil is.

History

The use of devices within the womb dates back to the last part of the nineteenth century. Those early devices looked rather like old-fashioned collar-studs and fitted into the cervical canal or entrance to the womb rather than within the actual cavity where a pregnancy would develop. It seems probable that these devices were also used to produce an abortion in women who were already pregnant.

It was not until 1909 that a Dr Richter in Germany first published any information about an intrauterine device in the medical literature. His device was in the form of a ring made of silk-worm gut, but this idea did not really catch on until 20 years later when Gräfenberg produced a ring of silk-worm gut surrounded by a substance called German Silver. German Silver is an alloy of copper, nickel, and zinc and it is interesting that since this time we have come to realize that copper and zinc may have a specific effect in preventing pregnancy.

The problem with these early ring-shaped devices was that they were not really flexible. They could only be put inside the wombs of women who had already had pregnancies and even then the entrance of the womb had to be stretched to put the device in. Because of these difficulties and because people suspected that there might be an association between the rings and infection within the womb, the intrauterine device developed no further in the following 30 years.

The plastic IUCD

However, in 1960 a new generation of devices was born with the advent of the Margulies spiral. By this time plastic technology had developed to the point where a device could be produced with a 'shape-memory'. This meant that a 'coil' of plastic could be temporarily straightened out or flattened in order to insert it into the womb. Once inside the cavity of the womb the device would spring back to its original shape. This advance meant that IUCDs could be inserted without first stretching up the entrance to the womb. The Margulies spiral was soon followed by the Lippes loop. This device, named after Dr Jack Lippes who designed it in 1962, is not truly a loop but more a crackerjack shape. It is still the most widely used IUCD in the world today, although, as we will discuss later in this chapter, it no longer has much place in Western society. Figure 8 shows some of the plastic IUCDs.

Following the introduction of these new flexible plastic devices many different shapes were designed and literally dozens of these are still available around the world. However, there were still problems with these second generation devices. First, they were so large that although they could be inserted at an out-patient appointment, they did not usually suit the woman who had not yet had any pregnancies. (The size of the cavity inside the womb increases after a woman's first pregnancy and thus accommodates this kind of coil more easily.) The second problem was that scientists discovered that the success of these devices depended on their surface area; thus the larger the device, the better it protected a woman against pregnancy. Unfortunately, the womb does not take kindly to

The intrauterine contraceptive device

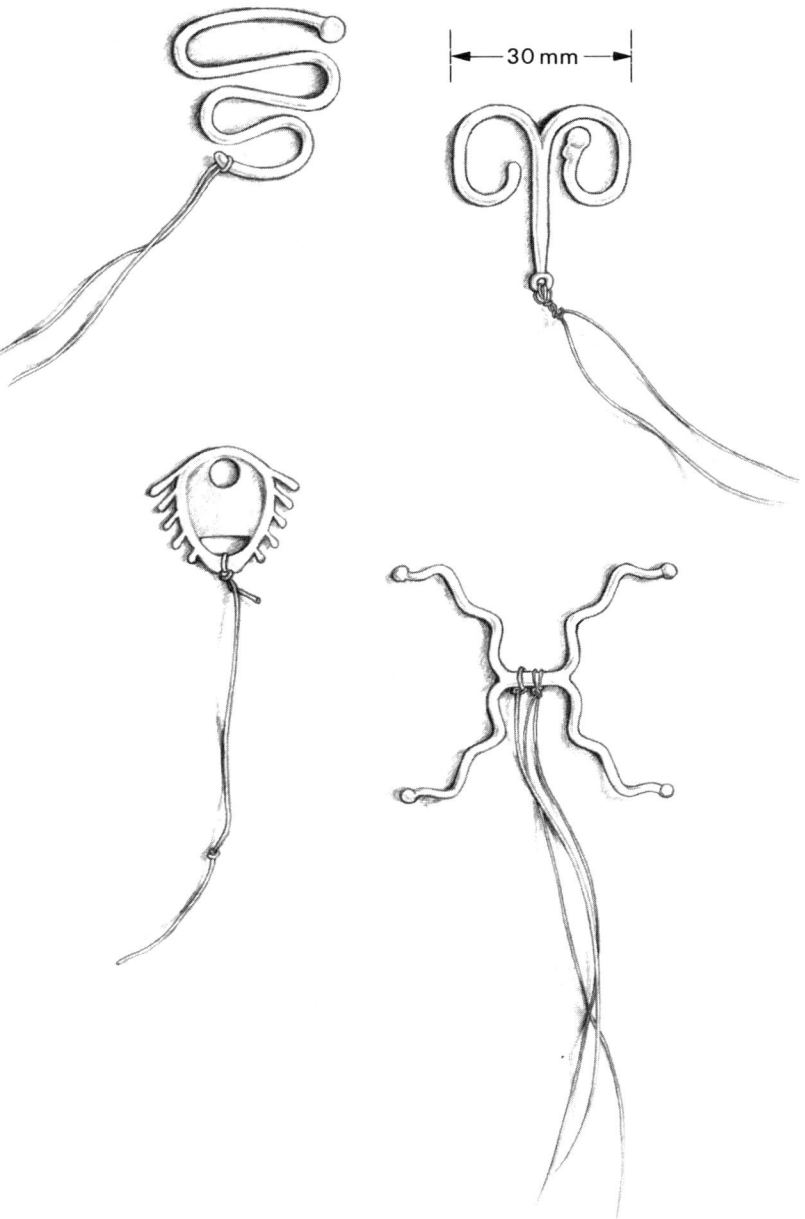

Fig. 8. Older IUCDs: plastic or inert type.

having foreign objects inside it, and the larger the device the more it complains. Thus IUCD designers had great difficulty finding a compromise between a device which was big enough to have a low failure rate while still giving an acceptably low rate of problems with discomfort and bleeding.

Medicated IUCDs

It was in response to this problem that the third generation or 'medicated' devices were designed. Though often called coils, these devices tend to be a totally different shape. They work on the principle that the plastic is just there to hold within the womb a chemical which will work to prevent pregnancy. Several chemicals have been tried, but the most successful of these have been copper and the hormone progesterone. In practice, most women who have IUCDs in this country today have a copper-bearing device. Fig. 9 shows some of the most commonly used copper IUCDs.

The copper gives the device a number of advantages. First, it makes it possible to use a much smaller piece of plastic. This makes the insertion of the IUCD easier and less uncomfortable. It also means that for the first time we have a number of IUCDs which can be used comfortably and safely by women who have never been pregnant and which are less likely to cause pain or bleeding from the womb. Perhaps even more importantly the copper IUCDs have been shown to have a lower pregnancy rate than previous generations of IUCDs.

How do you decide whether the IUCD is the right method for you? We will come back to this question later in this chapter, but perhaps first you need to know more about the advantages and disadvantages of the copper IUCD.

How the IUCD is fitted

In our experience one of the commonest factors preventing women from using the IUCD is the fear that it will be painful

The intrauterine contraceptive device

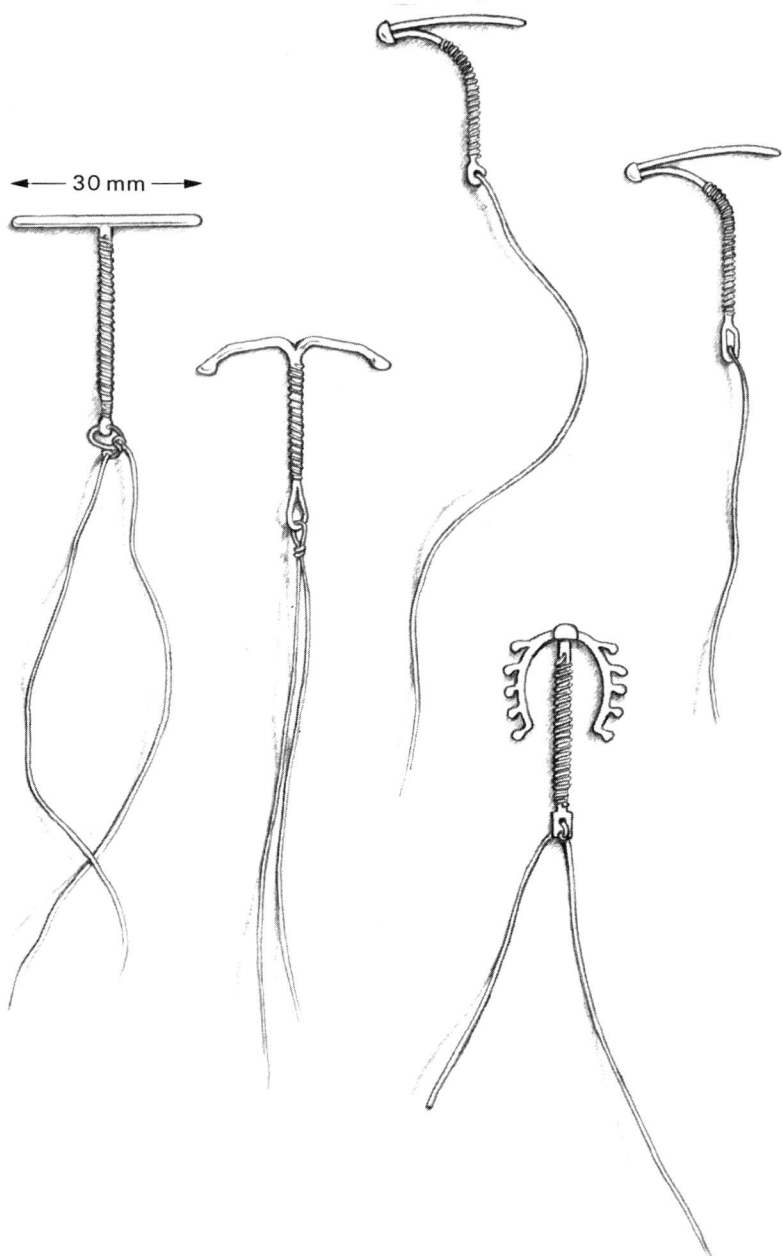

30 mm

Fig. 9. Newer IUCDs: all have copper wire around the stem.

to have one inserted. In fact, without exception our patients tell us afterwards that they are surprised at how easy it has been.

Most doctors suggest that if you are going to have an IUCD you should have it inserted during or just after the end of a period. This serves several purposes: first, at least you know that you are unlikely to be pregnant already. Secondly, and perhaps more importantly, the canal which leads from the top of the vagina into the womb opens up slightly during a period, thus making more room for the IUCD to be put in. It used to be believed that IUCDs would give less trouble if inserted at this time of the month, though not all doctors believe this now.

What is it like to have an IUCD inserted? The main problem is that the body's natural reaction to finding a strange object inside the womb is to try and push it out, and so almost everybody experiences some cramping of the womb muscle at the time of insertion. This cramping can often be blocked by anti-arthritis drugs like Ponstan which some clinics give before the insertion.

In order to insert the coil the doctor must first examine you internally. This is in order to check the size and position of the womb. A small metal instrument is then inserted into the vagina (in the same way as when you have a smear test). The neck of the womb is grasped with an instrument and this often gives a momentary sharp pinching feeling. The doctor then measures the distance from the womb entrance to the top of the cavity inside. The coil itself is then folded flat into a small tube called an introducer. The size of the coil inside an introducer is often narrower than the entrance into the womb, so the actual insertion of the IUCD will usually only cause a slight twinge of discomfort. The whole procedure takes less than a couple of minutes and, as we say, it is usually surprisingly painless.

The IUCD now lies within the cavity of the womb and hanging from it are one or two fine nylon threads which come through the neck of the womb into the top of the vagina. You can feel these threads yourself by inserting a finger well into the vagina, but they also serve as an easy way for removing the IUCD when required. Occasionally your partner may feel the threads during sex, but if he does the doctor can easily alter the length of the threads. It is usually suggested that a doctor or nurse should check the presence of these threads about six weeks after the IUCD is inserted, and then again once or twice a year.

How the IUCD works

At this point it would probably be appropriate for us to discuss how the IUCD works but, unfortunately, we only have limited information on this. It seems certain that the copper devices work in two main ways. First, they make it less likely that the sperms will be able to swim through the cavity of the womb to meet the egg; but their other, and more controversial, action is that if a sperm does meet an egg and conception takes place, the effect of the IUCD on the womb lining will prevent the fertilized egg from implanting and starting a pregnancy. This is a source of deep concern to many people, since although most scientists believe that pregnancy begins with the implantation of the fertilized egg into the wall of the womb, the teachings of some religions are that life begins when the sperm meets the egg. For those people the coil might be seen to be producing early abortions. For most, however, this argument seems academic and the IUCD is well accepted as a contraceptive.

Disadvantages

We have already implied that the copper IUCD is superior in most respects to the older devices, but this does not mean that it is without its snags. Clearly, its disadvantages will be more important to some women than to others.

Failure rate

Perhaps one of the more important drawbacks is the fact
that it does fail sometimes. Although it is not as reliable as
the pill, it does come a very good second and most modern
copper IUCDs have a failure rate of 1 to 2 per 100
woman-years. What this means in practice is that if we insert
100 IUCDs today, we expect to see one or two of those
women returning pregnant with each year that passes. For
those for whom even this rate is too high, it is possible to
make the IUCD safer still by using some additional
precautions (such as sperm-killing pessaries or foam) during
the most fertile time of the month (see Chapter 6).

Why does the IUCD fail? Sometimes it fails because it is
no longer there. As we have already said, the womb does
not take kindly to the presence of a foreign object and will
do its best to expel the IUCD, particularly during a period.
It is surprisingly easy not to notice this and that is the reason
why the thread or the threads on the device should be
checked from time to time, especially following the first
period after insertion. However, other IUCDs fail even
when they are still in the right place and this is the source of
another problem.

Effect on the fetus

Initially most people were worried about the possible effect
of an IUCD remaining within the womb during a pregnancy.
They were afraid that the copper, or even the mechanical
presence of the IUCD, might damage the developing baby.
However, we are now as sure as it is possible to be that there
is no such danger.

Miscarriage. On the other hand, what we do now realize is
that a pregnancy with an IUCD in the womb is much more
likely to end early. Although we do not know quite how
often pregnancies end in miscarriage, we think that probably
one in six fail to get past the first three months. For the

86

women with an IUCD in place, miscarriage may be much commoner, occurring in perhaps half of all cases where it is the first pregnancy. However, if the device is removed as soon as the woman is known to be pregnant then this danger is reduced. For this reason it is important for any woman using the IUCD to go to her doctor at the first suspicion of a pregnancy.

One might think that if the pregnancy were unwanted anyway one could leave the IUCD in place and hope for a miscarriage. Unfortunately, this is not a safe thing to do because the miscarriage can sometimes be infected (or 'septic') making the woman quite unwell.

Early labour. Sometimes, of course, it is not possible to remove the IUCD at the beginning of a pregnancy. As the womb grows so the IUCD and the thread with it may be carried up out of reach. If this does happen there is a slightly increased risk of going into labour early, but as we have said the woman can be reassured that there is no risk to the actual development of her baby.

Ectopic pregnancy. When we discussed the way in which the IUCD might be working, we said that it probably prevented the implantation of the fertilized egg on the wall of the womb. There has been a lot of discussion among the experts as to whether it also slows the journey of the egg down the tube into the womb. If we look at all pregnancies occurring in women with IUCDs then we find an increased proportion of these pregnancies are developing in the Fallopian tube rather than in the womb. This condition is called an ectopic pregnancy, and unless a woman seeks medical help early it can be quite dangerous. It can also result in loss of the tube in which the pregnancy is developing. There are two possible explanations for the increased proportion of these pregnancies in IUCD users. The pessimists feel that the IUCD actually makes ectopic pregnancies more frequent, but there is an alternative explanation. About one pregnancy in every 100 occurs in the tube, even in women using no contraception. If we assume that the IUCD offers good protection against a pregnancy occurring in the womb, but has no direct action on the egg while it is in the tube, then we would expect that IUCD 'failures' would include both those pregnancies in the womb which the IUCD had failed to prevent plus those occurring in the tube. This argument has not been completely resolved yet, but it is important for the woman with an IUCD, who misses a period, to know of the possibility of a tubal pregnancy. When this does occur it usually becomes apparent because of vaginal bleeding and pain in one or other of the bottom corners of the abdomen.

Effect on menstruation

Since the earliest days of the IUCD one of the main complaints about it has been its effect on the menstrual periods. Although the copper IUCDs affect the periods less than the old plastic-only devices, both increase the amount and duration of blood loss. The average woman with a coil probably loses about a quarter to one-third more during her period than she did before the coil was inserted. However, perhaps more annoyingly, the length of the period may also be increased. Typically, this is not an increase in the number of days of clear blood loss. Instead what happens is that a brownish discharge heralds the arrival of the period, but then continues for two or three days before true bleeding begins. At the other end of the period a similar tailing-off effect occurs, and the end result is that it is necessary to wear protection for longer than before. The only IUCD which has not produced this effect is the device which contains progesterone. This actually reduces the amount of menstrual loss, though it tends to cause a little light bleeding between the periods. Unfortunately, for a number of reasons these are not readily available in the United Kingdom.

The intrauterine contraceptive device

Infection

The last and most important association with the IUCD we would like to discuss is the increased tendency for IUCD users to get infection within the womb. We mentioned on p. 80 that the Gräfenberg ring fell into disrepute because of an apparent association with infection. Until recently a lot of family planning experts discounted this by saying that in fact infection within the womb was already common among the group of women who were using these early devices. However, over the last few years, a number of careful studies have been done and it is now clear that any woman with an IUCD is at increased risk for infection within the womb or the tubes. Different experts disagree about how much the risk is increased. It is probably about five times as common in IUCD users. It is important to realize that these increased risks of infection do not just apply to the promiscuous. The type of bacteria which we find within the womb in such cases are the sort which live normally in other parts of the body, such as the bowel, and so even the woman in the steadiest relationship may still be at risk. It seems from recent research that the thread hanging from the coil becomes covered in the natural secretions from the neck of the womb and provides a 'ladder' for the bacteria to climb up from the vagina into the womb.

We would not want to over-emphasize these risks of infection. It is important to understand that for most women this increased risk is still only 1 or 2 per cent. However, it is obviously important to know when you may have such an infection. Any woman using an IUCD who develops pain in the lower part of the abdomen combined with a temperature and an offensive discharge, should always go and see her doctor as soon as possible. Opinions about how best to treat an infection in an IUCD user have gone through a number of fashions. However, it now seems that the best plan is to start by taking some antibiotics. If the symptoms are not improving within 24 to 48 hours then it is probably worthwhile having the IUCD removed. We would suggest that anyone who has had a severe infection in the womb or tubes should have her IUCD removed and, if possible, should avoid having another for at least the following six months. The main problem with such infections is that unless they are treated promptly they can go on to cause discomfort and even to damage the tubes and affect fertility. Having said this, if we look at a large group of women who use the IUCD there is no evidence of any impairment of their fertility.

So far we have been discussing some of the unwanted side-effects of the IUCD. We hope this has not deterred you as it is important to remember that these problems only occur in a very small number of people and the vast majority of IUCD users find it a convenient, trouble-free method of contraception. After all, once an IUCD has been inserted there is nothing more to remember, and apart from the occasional check at the clinic contraception is no longer a problem.

How long IUCDs last

Unlike its bulkier, less effective predecessors the modern IUCD does not last for ever, and there has been much discussion among the experts about how long the copper devices can be considered to be effective. In the early 1970s when the first copper devices came on to the market it was advised that they should only be used for 18 months. This was then increased to two years, but then some evidence was obtained which suggested that they would not be so effective in a third year. Unfortunately, the methods underlying this research were faulty, and it is now known that all the copper IUCDs last a lot longer—probably for at least five or six years. However, there are two factors which limit their life-span. First, the copper is constantly dissolving. This is actually occurring at a very slow rate; so slow that we all eat more copper in a day's food than dissolves off an IUCD in the same time. The other factor affecting the life of the copper concerns the gradual cracking of the copper wire. This seems to occur more in some women than in others, but the copper can start to crack and small fragments then get washed away substantially shortening the life of the coil. To get around this one of the more recent devices, the Nova T, has a special wire made with a silver core surrounded by copper. This, of course, is more expensive to produce but it does mean that the device will last much longer, and it is already licensed for use for longer than any other copper-bearing IUCD. We are undoubtedly using all the copper coils for a lot less than their effective life-time, however, and doctors are gradually suggesting longer and longer periods between IUCD changes. This is important because every time an IUCD is replaced the woman has to go through a short 'settling-in' period when she can expect slightly more cramp from the womb as well as more bleeding between periods.

Reasons for not using an IUCD

We mentioned earlier the problem of how to decide whether the IUCD is the method for you. Perhaps we should discuss at this stage special conditions that may make the IUCD less suitable for certain women.

Heavy and painful periods

First, the woman who already has heavy or painful periods should be aware that these may get worse with an IUCD. Fortunately, we know enough about the causes of such period problems these days to be able to provide medicines which will reduce either the discomfort, or the amount of menstrual loss, or both. Obviously, though, having to use medicines to deal with the side-effects of your contraception is not ideal unless there are reasons for avoiding the other methods.

Infection

We have already discussed the problem of infection with IUCDs, and any woman who has had a serious infection within the womb, or who knows that her life-style places her at high risk of such infection, should avoid an IUCD if at all possible. The other group who should be cautious are those who have had rheumatic fever as children and are known to have had after-effects on their hearts. These women are at special risk for developing an infection in the valves of the heart, which can be triggered off by bacteria entering any other part of the body, and so for them the IUCD may present an extra hazard.

Sensitivity to copper

Another group that has been suggested as being at special risk with the IUCD is those who are known to be sensitive to copper, as it has been suggested that they might develop an allergic reaction to copper-bearing devices. As far as we know there is no objective evidence to support this idea.

Diabetes

Another group who have been warned off the IUCD in the past are diabetics. Some studies initially suggested that the IUCD might have a higher failure rate in women with diabetes and, of course, as well as this, diabetics are especially prone to infection. Recent studies, however, suggest that the copper IUCD works perfectly well in diabetics and there is no reason why they should be deterred from using this method.

The intrauterine contraceptive device

Summary

In summary, then, the modern copper-bearing IUCD provides a good method of contraception for some women. In its effectiveness it is second only to the pill. However, although it works locally rather than systemically like the pill, it has certain important side-effects. If it fails the resulting pregnancy may be in jeopardy unless the coil is removed early. The IUCD does not provide protection against pregnancy in the tube. It does affect most women's periods, usually making them somewhat heavier and longer. Lastly, there is a definite association between the IUCD and infection within the womb and tubes. On the positive side, however, once inserted it can be a trouble-free, reliable method of contraception which a woman can forget about apart from the occasional checks. It is ideal for the older woman who should not be taking the pill and for the woman who is delaying her next pregnancy. It is probably less suitable for the young girl who needs the minimum failure rate and cannot afford the associated risk of infection.

8

Post-coital contraception

Post-coital contraception arouses more feeling and emotion than almost any other method of contraception. It is not just that many people confuse it with abortion. It is not just the bad image that earlier drugs gave the method. It is not even the difficulty that many women have in getting to a clinic or their doctor the 'morning-after'. Many people, and not only doctors and nurses, dislike the idea of contraception after the event. Planned intercourse with planned contraception is acceptable, but being wise after the event is not. It would be melodramatic to say that they want to be able to control women's sexuality, but they manage to give that impression by expressing fears that women might make the same mistake more than once. Another fear that they have is that knowing that a back-up method is available might make consumers less likely to stick with their present method, and so 'live dangerously'. This is a similar argument to the one put forward by those who opposed seat-belt legislation on the grounds that it would encourage bad driving.

History

The history of post-coital contraception parallels that of contraception. From the earliest times after the link between intercourse and subsequent pregnancy was established, drugs, spells, and other manoeuvres were tried. Some of these were pure superstition, while others depended on a faulty knowledge of physiology. Some had a small degree of effectiveness. It is worth repeating though that humans in general are an infertile race. On the most fertile day of her cycle a woman has only a 1 in 4 chance of conceiving a child if she has intercourse with a fertile man—and the risk falls to less than 1 in 30 on the least fertile day. So any form of treatment—or nothing at all—will work on at least three occasions out of four. This keeps a lot of unscientific and inadequate methods alive in the mythology of old wives' tales.

Fallacies

Some facts need to be made clear at the start of this section.
1. An orgasm is not necessary for either successful transport of sperm in women, or for fertilization.
2. Douching, or washing out the vagina, is relatively ineffective at removing sperms because they leave the seminal fluid to swim into mucus which lines the cervix within a few minutes of being deposited there.
3. Those methods that hope to provide help after implantation has occurred are equally unreliable. However, one pregnancy in four or six will not come to term and, with all other things being equal, unwanted pregnancies have a higher spontaneous loss rate than wanted pregnancies. Some medicines will appear to work for some women occasionally. There are no drugs readily available that will cause a pregnancy that has already implanted to be expelled from the uterus, apart from those that are marketed solely for the purpose of producing abortions.

Early methods of post-coital contraception grew up from a misunderstanding of these facts. Women were instructed to drink a glass of cold water, or sneeze three times, or leap from the bed to perform calisthenics. More medical methods used douching. It is possible that the widespread use of the bidet in continental Europe, with its emphasis on vulval hygiene, related more to douching to try and prevent pregnancy than to worries about personal hygiene. Vaginal douches have been in use for many centuries, with recipes being found in the medical records of almost every culture. In recent years there have been claims—never backed up with evidence—that fizzy soft drinks like Coca-Cola have been used in Third World countries and the campuses of American universities as a contraceptive douche.

Modern methods of post-coital contraception

Modern methods depend on the understanding we now have of the hormonal events surrounding ovulation and conception. Drugs can be given in the hope of preventing ovulation and implantation, and the first ones began to be described in the mid-1920s. Unfortunately, the high incidence of side-effects, coupled with their lack of absolute effectiveness, lead to their under-use. Despite this, the need for them was so great that in a few pioneering centres many thousands of women were treated.

Post-coital contraception began to become important and more widely used in the early 1970s. Several factors were responsible for this. Two new developments made treatment easier, safer, more effective, and with fewer side-effects. A trend away from medical methods meant that some women were relying on less effective methods, or nothing at all, often after many years of relying on the pill. In addition, open discussion about some of the problems of sexuality meant that more people were getting the opportunity to find out about the availability of this type of service.

Modern post-coital contraception really began with the publication of the research of three men in New York in 1972. They were all eminent in the field of contraception, and more particularly in the field of intra-uterine contraception. They studied the effectiveness of a copper-containing IUCD that was inserted after unprotected intercourse, and found it to be very effective in preventing pregnancy. In their skilled hands there were very few other problems.

The next breakthrough occurred when a Canadian researcher tried the use of the pill when women had been exposed to the risk of pregnancy. Early trials were promising, and after the dose had been increased and more trials carried out, it became the standard method of treatment. However, the field has continued to expand. There have been three further refinements: the use of progestogen-only pills, the development of a low-dose oestrogen compound that can be injected (for women who are intolerant of oral drugs), and the use of Danazol (a drug more usually used to 'switch off' ovulation).

The IUCD

To go back to the first of the modern methods. The IUCD almost certainly acts by preventing the implantation of a fertilized egg. This event occurs about five days after fertilization, which in turn can occur anything from a few hours to a few days after intercourse. The effect of the device is immediate, and is probably greatest in the first few days after it has been inserted. We have already outlined the advantages and disadvantages of the device when used generally in contraception, but there are a few extra factors associated with its use in these circumstances.

Disadvantages. The device needs to be inserted by some-one with skill, and this skill might not be readily available every day. All devices can be painful to fit and, while not all fittings are painful, they can certainly be difficult for both the woman and her doctor. A well-prepared woman who has made a conscious decision and effort to have a device fitted may be able to cope with this, while someone who is upset following a recent contraceptive accident, or rape, may not be able to tolerate the insertion. Similarly, someone who has just had her first ever sexual encounter will probably not be able to relax sufficiently to enable the doctor to examine her and fit the device easily. In addition, infections are a known complication of the IUCD, and someone who may be in the early stages of a pelvic infection is at much greater risk of complications.

Advantages. The story is not all bad, though. Once the device is in place it will provide contraception until it is removed. This might mean the time of the next period, or it might be several years later. It is also one of the most effective methods of morning-after contraception. While an exact failure rate has not been calculated, it is probably less than one woman in every 1000 exposed to the risk of pregnancy.

Most women do not choose it as the best method for them. In Birmingham we carried out an experiment in which we offered those women who came to our clinic the choice of a post-coital IUCD or tablets. Almost all of them chose the tablets: very few were happy with the idea of an IUCD. They were worried about almost every aspect of the device but, more importantly, they were attracted by the simplicity and ease of the tablets.

The combined pill

There is really only one choice when it comes to oral post-coital contraception. Four tablets of Ovran, or Eugynon 50, when taken within three days of unprotected intercourse, will prevent pregnancy in nearly all of the women who take them. Because many of the women get feelings of nausea, or even start to vomit, it is usual to take the tablets in two doses of two tablets each, taken twelve hours apart. This does not seem to change the effectiveness of the pills, and leads to far fewer side-effects. Taking these four tablets within three days of intercourse is not as effective as fitting an IUCD but is much simpler, cheaper, and easier.

Side-effects. Side-effects are as common with these tablets as with the older high dose methods, but are not nearly as severe. Perhaps half of all users will complain of nausea and

98

sickness, and as many as a third will suffer from breast tenderness. Some of the earlier treatments needed the women to come into hospital to have their sickness and vomiting treated, but this does not happen with the four oral contraceptive tablet treatment we have just discussed. Most women say it affects their next period, usually by bringing it forward by a few days. In others it leads to a delay of a few days, and in a few instances it becomes more painful. The worrisome complications of the oestrogen-containing oral contraceptives on blood clotting and the heart and blood-vessels have not been reported. This is probably because these tablets are given in relatively small doses for very short periods of time.

Failure rate. The price paid for this ease of use is decreased effectiveness in preventing pregnancy. While women who have not been treated could expect to become pregnant about once in every four times they take a chance at ovulation time, the pregnancy rate for the four tablet treatment course is about one woman in every hundred treated. As we mentioned earlier, the rate for those women treated with copper-containing IUCDs is about one in every thousand treated.

What happens to the fetus if the pill fails? What happens to these pregnancies? Most of them are unplanned and not wanted. There are also not very many of them and, since most of them end up as abortions, there are not very many facts to go on. What facts there are suggest that those that are not terminated progress to term and continue much as any other pregnancy. There does not seem to be any evidence that they are any better or worse than any other unwanted pregnancies. This is important to remember, because many women who have no objection to taking morning-after contraception do have deep objections to abortion. Should the method fail for them they will want reassurance that they have not harmed their baby, and we feel able to give this to them. Many of the worries about giving hormones to pregnant women stem from the use of a drug called diethyl-stilboestrol that was once used to try and treat women who seemed unable to carry pregnancies to term. It has now been recognized as producing many abnormalities in children whose mothers were treated with it, although the abnormalities did not come to light until many years after the children had been born. These problems only seem to happen when high doses of drugs are given to women with well-established pregnancies. When the same drug was given as a post-coital contraceptive these problems were not reported.

How the pill works.   We still do not know how these drugs work. We understand some of the ways in which they act. They thicken the mucus at the neck of the womb, making it harder for spermatozoa to survive there. They act to delay the surge of hormones that release the eggs from the ovary and so, if given a few days before ovulation, they will delay or prevent the release of an egg. They might interfere with the way in which the Fallopian tubes contract, and so act to stop spermatozoa and eggs from meeting. Their most important action is to interfere with the sites on the cells that line the womb that respond to hormones. Hormones act on these cells rather like the way in which keys unlock doors. If a lock has been jammed by a misshapen key then no other key can open the door.

A fertilized egg will reach the womb a few days after fertilization. No-one knows how it burrows into the womb lining and starts to grow inwards. It is a very delicate, easily upset process, and if the cells that normally respond to the presence of the egg have their mechanisms for responding to the egg blocked by the pill hormones they will probably not accept and respond to the new hormone source. Many drugs interfere with the hormone-receptor sites, and some of these have been tried as post-coital contraceptives.

Post-coital contraception

Danazol

Danazol is one drug used as a post-coital contraceptive. It has been used for many years to 'switch off' ovulation, to help in the treatment of breast disease, heavy periods, premenstrual tension, and other similar conditions. Its use as a post-coital contraceptive is still new and experimental, and while it is unlikely to be more than an adjunct to therapy with oral contraceptives, it does provide research scientists with another tool to study the mechanisms of implantation of the egg into the womb.

Progestogens

We discussed progestogens in Chapters 4 and 5. The same forms of the same drugs are also used as post-coital contraceptives, but in higher doses than are used in either the combined pill or the progesterone-only pill. In addition, there have been some trials with other progestogens which have also been effective. One country where they seem to be successful when used on a regular basis is Peru. They have been used there by couples who spend large parts of the year apart and only meet at irregular intervals. High in the Andes communications are poor and husbands are unable to let wives know in advance of their return home. The women take post-coital progestogens for those occasions when their men are at home, seeing little sense in using contraceptives regularly when the need is infrequent.

Injectable oestrogens

A variation on the theme is the use of injectable oestrogens that has been tried in West Germany. The idea is to use a preparation broadly similar to the oral contraceptive, but in an injectable form. This means that women who vomit after taking the medicines need not worry about losing a dose. However, this sort of reaction does not happen very often and the method will probably not be widely used. Most women seem to prefer the simplicity of the four-tablet treatment plan.

Reasons for using post-coital contraception

So far we have talked more about the methods themselves than the people who might want to use them. Far more important than any contraceptive method is its availability, and the wish of people to use it. More unwanted pregnancies can be prevented by methods that people will find acceptable rather than by theoretically better methods that they dislike or cannot be bothered to use.

In the early days of 'morning-after' contraception it really was just as the name implies—a few women used the method after unprotected intercourse had occurred. It was only ever used as an emergency method. There is now a trend for it to be offered right from the start as a back-up for other methods, and our study in Birmingham was one of the first to show this!

Failure of the condom

A small proportion of couples use the sheath as a contraceptive. These are frequently couples who do not want a pregnancy at all. Many of them have had to stop using the pill because of medical problems, or the worry that they might have because of the wife's increasing age, and they do not want a pregnancy at any cost. Recent studies on the usage of post-coital contraception say that the majority of users, often as many as two-thirds of the total, request help following a sheath breakage. Many of the couples who find that a sheath has broken during intercourse are unused to this method of contraception and were careless in putting it on, or started intercourse before the woman was properly lubricated. Some are experienced sheath users, and for the first time in perhaps years of use have had an accident.

Post-coital contraception

Using no contraception

A smaller number of requests come from those who had not intended to have intercourse, but had got 'carried away'. It is worth remembering that two-thirds of people use no contraception when they have intercourse for the first ever time. It takes little effort to realize why this is so—the decision to lose virginity is rarely a conscious one, and for most people is a spontaneous event. It is only rarely a planned event that can be anticipated.

Availability

In the early days of the use of post-coital contraception it was difficult to find supplies. In the United Kingdom all contraception was ignored by many family doctors for many years, and it is only in the last decade that the majority have begun to see it as part of their overall care of families. Until recently many family planning clinics were open only at irregular times, and used appointment systems. This restricted the availability of emergency contraception and meant that those women who had heard about the possibilities of such treatment were often frustrated by the seeming impossibility of getting it!

It is possible now to get the tablets from most family doctors, most of whom will see women with this kind of emergency as soon as they possibly can. If women are unwilling or unable to see their own doctors then organizations in Britain like the British Pregnancy Advisory Service, or the Brook Clinics, will usually have a walk-in service to provide assistance. Most Family Planning or Planned Parenthood clinics, while still not open every day, will provide help, and it is usually possible to find an open clinic within the three days deadline for the use of pills. Unfortunately many clinics close over holiday periods. In parts of the United Kingdom the Pregnancy Advisory Services or

BPAS use telephone answering services to give advice about the availability of help outside of normal hours.

The future

It is against this background that we should see the future of post-coital contraception. As an emergency method most people will only need it once. Unless they are made aware of its existence the opportunity to use it may be lost, and they might be faced with an unwanted pregnancy. Any advertising campaign needs to be sustained and obvious. In the United Kingdom most of the advertising comes from the private and charitable sector, and they are restricted to small inserts in the personal section of the classified advertisements in newspapers and magazines. The huge posters on the sides of buses that advertise life insurance are not permitted as appropriate for this type of personal help!

Another part of the future for post-coital contraception is in the deliberate provision of help for self-medication in people at risk. Some family planning authorities are at present debating a suggestion to allow the supply of packets of condoms which will include a separate insert of four post-coital tablets. These could be used by women if the sheath slipped off or tore. While many authorities see the sense in this, others dislike the move to self-medication and loss of control over prescription-only medicines.

9

Natural methods of family planning

We have discussed so far many different methods of reversible contraception, all of which involve men wearing condoms, or women taking drugs, or being fitted with IUCDs or barriers. There are other forms of contraception that are possibly more widespread than any of these methods. Natural methods of family planning prevent pregnancy without the use of chemical agents or physical devices. They are as old as recorded history and probably almost universally used. They include variants on the barrier methods, but instead of physical barriers use barriers in space and time, or utilize the natural antifertility effect of breast-feeding.

History

The first recorded user of a natural method is Onan who, in Genesis, is reported as spilling his seed to prevent his brother's wife from becoming pregnant. This has been taken to mean that he practised coitus interruptus, or withdrawal. He was punished for this but many men still follow his example. Mohammed did not allow his followers to use coitus interruptus if the woman did not consent to it. He is credited in the post-Koranic writings with saying 'Had it been injurous it would have harmed the Romans and the Persians'. Most people have on at least one occasion in their lives practised one of the natural methods. There are now far fewer couples in the West who use only withdrawal as a means of contraception than there were fifteen years ago, and even fewer who use the 'rhythm' method. The wider availability of newer methods of contraception and the fact that all contraception is now more openly discussed has led to the 'non-natural' methods superseding coitus interruptus and similar methods.

Over the past few years—in response to the realization that more people were using artificial methods of pregnancy control—the Catholic church has assisted in putting a newer face on to the rhythm method. It is now called Natural Family Planning and we discuss it much more fully later in the chapter. At the same time, the growing ecological movement with a back-to-nature element has meant that some young people do not want to use synthetic methods, and many women want to experience ovulation and avoid pregnancy by avoiding vaginal sexual contact at the time they are at greatest risk of pregnancy. These trends have led to a reappraisal of natural methods, with an attempt to put them on to a firmer scientific footing.

One other important natural method that has been talked about more in recent years is breast-feeding. A few years ago it was estimated that breast-feeding was preventing more pregnancies throughout the world than all other methods of contraception put together. This relative importance has declined over the past decade because world-wide women are not breast-feeding for so long, while at the same time other methods of contraception are becoming more easily available. One problem with breast-feeding as a contraceptive method, as we shall discuss later, is that although it is very effective on a population level, its effectiveness at an individual level is debatable.

In this chapter we shall discuss the three main natural methods in turn. The first methods—those which seek to put a natural physical barrier between the egg and sperm—need little introduction. The second group, periodic abstinence, the rhythm method, or 'natural family planning,' are variations on the theme of putting a barrier in time between the egg and the sperm, while breast-feeding relies for its effectiveness on the natural switching off of ovulation that occurs when the hormone prolactin is secreted in response to nipple stimulation. The last section of the chapter will attempt to put natural methods into their historical perspective.

Natural barriers between egg and sperm

Pregnancy prevention by the use of natural physical barriers can either be achieved by withdrawing the penis before ejaculation, or making sure that there is no contact between the vagina and the penis from the start of sexual activity. A recent estimate in the United Kingdom suggested that in the years 1967–68 (less than a decade after the introduction of the pill) coitus interruptus was used, or had been used at some stage, by 27 per cent of professional people and about 53 per cent of blue-collar families. In the survey carried out in Britain in 1976 that we discussed in Chapter 2, only 6 per cent of couples were still using this method.

There are no figures available for the proportion of people using each of the different methods of non-vaginal ejaculation, but the consensus of opinion is that the commonest method is withdrawal, with very few couples using coitus intra-crura (intercourse between the thighs) or non-vaginal sexual activity. Some couples combine non-vaginal sexual activity, which is principally oral or anal sex, with periodic abstinence. They will reserve vaginal intercourse for those parts of the cycle when conception is unlikely to occur.

One rarely mentioned advantage of these methods is that to be successful much more communication is needed between couples than is customary in many relationships. They need to discuss the position they will use, so that the woman can contribute to the success as much as the man. Many couples find the 'spoon' position the most successful. In this position the man enters his partner from behind. He is able to stimulate her breasts and clitoris and, in addition, men are unable to achieve deep penetration because of the mechanical disadvantage they are at. Withdrawal is easier, and the fact that the labia close after withdrawal of the penis tends to keep semen outside the vagina rather than letting it leak in. Some couples find that they can prolong their pleasure by using the 'squeeze' technique. This technique was popularized by the American sex researchers Masters and Johnson, to deal with the treatment of premature ejaculation. It requires almost perfect communication between partners since the aim is to squeeze the base of the glans of the penis when ejaculation is close. If it is left too late then ejaculation becomes inevitable, and if it is performed too soon then it is ineffective. For some couples the extra pleasure they get from these techniques goes some way to compensating for the lack of absolute effectiveness of the methods.

Despite the drawback of a relatively high failure rate, these methods have been used and will continue to be used by many couples. Failure rates are almost impossible to establish, since very few couples register at family planning clinics to use this method and so estimates tend to be based on broader sociological surveys. It has been suggested that for every hundred couples using this method for a year there will be between 5 and 15 pregnancies. Doctors and nurses get a biased view of those who use these methods since they either see the failures—those who have become pregnant—or those who are unhappy with the method and are seen at clinics asking for a change. Most couples use these methods without coming to the attention of the medical profession. For successful couples these methods have the advantage of being easy to use and not needing medical supervision.

An important contribution that the advocates of natural methods of family planning have made is to show that success with these methods depends on the counselling, teaching, and support of the couples involved. Almost every study that has been undertaken has shown that success in avoiding pregnancy is better in those who want to stop pregnancies, rather than merely delaying their next one, and it is better also in those who have support over a long period of time. Women whose information is limited to a few lectures, or is straight from books, tend either to abandon the method or to become pregnant. Unfortunately, the teaching and long-term support needed for these methods to be successful is very labour-intensive, and there is a shortage of dedicated and skilled teachers.

The teaching methods involve three main phases. The first is where you, your partner, and your counsellor build up a rapport. This is important because you are going to be asked in the second phase to identify ovulation and you may be unsure of your own anatomy and physiology and need a lot of help from the counsellor to determine this. You will then have to have one of your most private activities held up to scrutiny and prohibited for a large part of each month. This prohibition can be for as long as two-and-a-half weeks in each month for some couples. There are many ways of pinpointing the safe time in each month and once you have chosen the method, or better still the combination of methods, that you are going to use, you will be carefully schooled in its practical aspects. The third phase involves the sexual counselling which is necessary because these methods can be stressful. Not only does the ban on sexual activity create problems, but occasional lapses can create feelings of guilt and inadequacy. Supporting couples through these difficulties is one of the roles of the counsellors, and much effort is at present being directed at the training of them. The World Health Organization in particular has several training and evaluation programmes. It should be emphasized that the prohibitions are on vaginal sexual activity only—other forms of mutual pleasure-giving are not only allowed but encouraged.

'Rhythm method'

To detect ovulation you need to know the changes that occur in the body during the monthly ovarian cycle. In the early part of the cycle there is a gradual build-up of the mucus at the neck of the womb to accommodate and protect the sperms. At the same time, recognizable changes occur in the tissues of the cervix and you can learn to recognize the change in texture. Ovulation itself is accompanied by a sharp pain in some women, and the release of the hormone progesterone from the ovary after the release of the egg is accompanied by changes in the mucus, the cervix, and a rise in temperature of 1 °F or ½ °C. Ovulation tends to occur about 14 days before the next period begins, and so if you have regular periods the date of ovulation can be predicted. It is this inherent rhythmicity that led to the old term of 'the rhythm method'.

It is customary to divide the monthly cycle into three phases—the pre-ovulatory infertile phase, the ovulatory fertile phase, and the post-ovulatory infertile phase. In practice, of course, there is no clear distinction between the three phases, and so to avoid any risk of pregnancy most couples extend the arbitrary length of the fertile phase at the expense of the two phases of relative infertility. It is also important to realize that in many women cervical mucus starts being produced many days before ovulation, and can sometimes keep sperms alive for many days. Nobody is sure for how long sperms can retain their ability to fertilize an egg. Many people have reported seeing active sperm in the cervical mucus one week after they were put there, but it is possible that although the sperm were still alive they did not have the ability to swim up through the genital tract to the egg and to fertilize it. We discuss later in the chapter the concern that some doctors have about the effect of these ageing sperms on a potential pregnancy.

The pre-ovulatory infertile phase

The pre-ovulatory infertile period is not as easy to recognize as the post-ovulatory one. It extends from the beginning of menstruation to the first appearance of the cervical mucus which can keep sperms alive. If the calendar method is being used then this is about 18 days before the next period but, because of the variability most women experience, the calendar method alone is not precise enough. In addition, because of the way that cervical mucus protects and nourishes spermatozoa, merely using the dates of the last few periods is not sufficiently reliable as there can be enough mucus present several days before the expected date of ovulation to keep sperm alive. This difficulty in defining the pre-ovulatory infertile period is one of the principal sources of error for this technique. There are two main ways of overcoming it—either abstaining from intercourse for the first part of the cycle, and having intercourse only during the more clearly defined post-ovulatory period, or using additional methods to diagnose the pre-ovulatory infertile period.

The Australian husband and wife family planning team of Billings and Billings made one of the great contributions to this subject when they studied the interrelationships between the look and feel of cervical mucus and fertility. The study of many thousands of cycles, by them and others, has shown that intercourse before the surge of ovarian hormones which produces cervical mucus does not lead to pregnancy. They have shown that if women can be taught to recognize the presence of cervical mucus they will know when to stop having sex. Women are taught to observe their mucus patterns at the vulva, relying on the sensation of wetness and lubrication that the mucus produces. The mucus becomes clearer, more profuse, and stretchier as ovulation approaches. This is called the build-up phase and leads to the 'peak' symptom which occurs on the last day that this type of mucus is produced. Ovulation is thought to occur very close to this time. The pre-ovulatory infertile phase ends on the first day that mucus secretion begins.

You will be taught not only how to examine yourself to feel your cervix and collect mucus from it, but also how to distinguish it from normal and abnormal vaginal fluids. The likeliest sources of vaginal fluid are the normal discharge after intercourse and the lubricating fluid produced in response to sexual arousal. These can both be distinguished from cervical mucus, but because this is quite difficult some teachers say that in the first part of the cycle couples should not have any sort of sexual activity more than once every two to three days, because if they have it more often they can interfere with the mucus signs and this can lead to pregnancy.

The ovulatory fertile period

The ovulatory fertile period is said to begin on the first day that mucus is produced, and to end four clear days after the 'peak' mucus symptom. Obviously women are not fertile for all of that time, because the egg only lives for a few hours and probably less than one day. In addition, it is quite probable that spermatozoa can only survive and be effective for a few days.

The extra days at either end of the period are to try and increase the method's effectiveness. In some women ovulation itself produces recognizable symptoms. The most famous one is *Mittelschmerz* or ovulation pain. It is rarely translated from the original German because there is no direct English counterpart, but it means 'mid-cycle pain'. It refers to the sharp pain that some women get in their lower abdomen at around the time of ovulation.

Mittelschmerz pain begins about 12 hours before ovulation. The cause for it is not known but it might be related to the stretching of the skin around the ovary as the developing egg begins to swell before being released. It may occur on only one side, with no pain being produced in months when the ovary on the other side is releasing an egg. Some women do not feel it but can produce it by bouncing up and down suddenly on a firm surface, like a hard chair. This will often, if they are near ovulation, produce a sharp pain that is characteristic of ovulation.

There are some drawbacks for couples using the ovulation-detection method. They have to abstain from intercourse during menstruation, because some women might produce mucus then and not notice it. This means that any bleeding between periods can also stop them from having intercourse, both on the days of bleeding and for the next three days (since small amounts of blood can have quite an effect on the mucus).

All of these natural methods have disadvantages. The restrictions on intercourse can lead to disharmony between couples, unless they are better at communicating in other ways than most are, or have a very experienced counsellor assisting them. None is absolutely fool-proof, and while failure rates of only 2 per cent per year and less have been reported for dedicated couples with the support of good centres, there is still a substantial risk for ordinary couples. Failure rates of more than 20 per cent per year have come from some studies, including some carefully controlled ones carried out by the World Health Organization.

The post-ovulatory infertile period

To try and reduce the risks of pregnancy some teachers will encourage couples to restrict intercourse to the well-defined, and safe, post-ovulatory infertile period. This starts at the end of the fertile phase and ends at the beginning of menstruation. It is characterized by two main features, both related to the release of the hormone progesterone from the ovary after the egg has been released. As soon as progesterone is secreted into the bloodstream it begins to dry up the mucus from the neck of the womb and changes it into a barrier to sperm once again. It is no longer slippery, and when stretched apart on the fingers will not stretch more than half-an-inch, or about one centimetre. It is also cloudy and scanty. Progesterone also affects the temperature of the

113

body. This goes up by about 1 °F (about 0·5 °C) within a day of the release of the egg. This is one of the surest ways of confirming ovulation, but, because a woman's temperature can rise for many reasons other than ovulation, most people say that to be sure a temperature rise is caused by ovulation and not just a random fluctuation, there is a risk of pregnancy until the temperature has been up for three days. It does not matter how or when the temperature is taken provided it is always taken at the same time of day and from the same place in the body. The commonest time to take the temperature is early morning, but many women prefer to do it at bed-time or in the early evening. There are certain obvious provisos—no hot meals or drinks, or cigarettes, in the hours before the temperature is taken. Similarly, while most women are happy to slip the thermometer under their tongues, some will want to take their temperature rectally (because that is a better indicator of the inner body temperature) or vaginally (because that shares the same advantages as the rectal temperature whilst at the same time being near the ovaries, which may or may not be a good thing). Whatever you decide to do, you should use the same method each time.

All of these difficulties with pinpointing ovulation and avoiding mucus means that the most effective method of periodic abstinence is to prohibit intercourse for all of the month except the period from three days after ovulation until menstruation. For many couples this means that they can make love for only 10 days in each month, which is difficult for many, not only those who are in the throes of a new relationship.

Periodic abstinence has many advantages as a method of contraception. For individual couples it is cheap (although it is labour-intensive with a lot of counselling, teaching, and support needed, but fortunately these are usually provided by lay workers, motivated by zeal rather than financial inducements). Its proponents say that it is safe, avoiding the hazards of chemical contraception and the IUCD. Its opponents say the method is ineffective, applying the fairly derisory title of 'Vatican roulette'. It is worth looking in greater detail at these claims and counter-claims.

Disadvantages

There is no doubt that these methods avoid the known hazards of oral contraception. However, as we saw in those chapters, oral contraception, especially using the combined pill, produces many benefits as well as having a small, but finite, risk to health from the oestrogens. Women who take these drugs have a significantly reduced incidence of cancer of the lining of the womb and they suffer from fewer cancerous and non-cancerous cysts of the ovary. They suffer from less breast disease, with fewer lumps that need medical attention. There is less rheumatoid arthritis among those women who take them, and there is of course almost complete freedom from pregnancy with much greater freedom of sexual expression. These advantages do not of course apply to those who use periodic abstinence as a method of contraception, but there is an additional anxiety that some doctors have about the use of this method.

As with almost all other contraceptive measures, these methods share the problem of abnormal development of a pregnancy which may result from a contraceptive failure. While the IUCD and the progestogen-only pill may be linked with ectopic pregnancy, periodic abstinence and spermicides are linked with spontaneous abortion and fetal maldevelopment. It is not known if the mechanisms are the same. It might be that periodic abstinence allows a much greater chance of an aged sperm fertilizing an egg, or an aged egg meeting a spermatozoon. It is unlikely that the process of death and decay of either sperms or eggs is sudden, and it is much more likely that there is a loss of the ability to develop normally over a period of several hours. It may be that it is this sort of ageing egg that is more likely to have abnormal genetic development. These abnormalities show themselves as either miscarriages or chromosomally abnormal babies. The last occurrence is very rare, and still contentious, with different scientists giving different views. It is probably for the best that very little research has been done on this last potential hazard. There is so much guilt and anguish surrounding the birth of an abnormal baby that to start attributing it to a failure of a contraceptive method, that some people feel morally obliged to use, is inhumane.

One point that was popular with the press some years ago is the theory that failures of this method are more, or sometimes less, likely to be boys. Unfortunately, there is no foundation for this belief either. Nobody has yet found a method of selecting the sex of a baby before conception, although this lack of success has not stopped people from trying.

It has been suggested that since, in Western Europe at least, Catholics use the same methods of contraception as their counterparts in other faiths, those who use periodic abstinence are those who are prepared to put up with the restrictions on intercourse, while others with higher sex drives have moved on to methods like the pill or the IUCD.

Breast-feeding

A decade ago it was estimated that breast-feeding was preventing more pregnancies throughout the world than all other methods put together. As a contraceptive measure it has been ranked second only to the combined pill in effectiveness, but there is still much argument about this. It is certainly effective on a global scale but there is still some debate about its effectiveness for individual women.

When a baby sucks from the breast there is a reflex release of the hormone prolactin from the pituitary gland at the base of the brain. This hormone acts primarily on the breast to help produce more milk but it also has two subsidiary effects. The first is to prevent the release of the hormones from the pituitary that act on the ovary to start ovulation, but there is also a direct action on the ovary to stop ovulation. Laboratory tests have shown that prolactin will also act directly on the cells in the ovary that secrete progesterone and stop the secretion of this hormone. The significance of this in real life is not clear.

Prolactin does not last for very long in the bloodstream. Half of the prolactin that has been released in a burst following suckling is broken down by the body is less than 30 minutes. This means that although the amount of hormone released into the bloodstream at least doubles, and often rises 20-fold within a few minutes of the start of suckling, this effect is short-lived. Therefore, the effect on ovulation is intermittent, and a woman who breast-feeds only a few times a day has normal prolactin levels for most of the day. This might not be very important if prolactin acts on the cells of the ovary which produce progesterone since this might prevent the development of any eggs which have been released. This is still not proven.

The most important factor is that, to keep the levels of prolactin high enough for there to be a reliable anti-fertility effect, nipple stimulation by suckling needs to be regularly repeated throughout the day. This is not practicable in Western societies, where the practice is that even 'demand-fed' babies will only feed on about six or seven occasions each day, with many babies (especially the good ones!) going throughout the night without waking and demanding to be fed.

There is evidence that until comparatively recently man has been primarily a hunter–gatherer, with most societies consisting of nomadic wanderers. Settled populations of villages only began to appear about 10 000 years ago. This means that most of human evolution has been aimed at the nomadic existence, with few adaptations having appeared yet for city life. There are now very few hunter–gatherer societies left, but a group which has been extensively studied are the !Kung bushmen of the Kalahari desert. They are not a typical African society because they live in the desert, where they live a nomadic existence. Despite the fact that they live in an extremely harsh environment there is no evidence they are malnourished, apart from some mild seasonal reduction in calories. (They are much smaller in stature than similar African tribes and this may well be related to food deprivation during the growing years of childhood.) They are a very pro-birth society, where families aim to have as many children as possible, and yet despite this women have on average less than five children. Unlike many other non-Westernized societies, they do not believe in sexual continence during lactation, and the wife does not leave her husband to live with her parents during the early years of child-rearing.

Contraception for these women seems to be almost entirely achieved by the anti-ovulatory effects of breast-feeding. They do not feed their babies in the Western tradition but instead keep their babies with them for most of the day and night. Several anthropologists have reported that it is rare for a baby, or child under the age of two, to be away from the breast for more than 15 minutes, and this seems to happen (though possibly not with the same frequency) even during the night.

The effects of this sort of intensive, long-term raising of the blood prolactin level is to switch off ovarian function for many years. The average !Kung woman has a space of three to four years between pregnancies, and might only have a dozen menstrual periods in her entire life. During this time she will have, on average, between four and five children.

The absence of ovulation for such a long period seems to have one big advantage and one big disadvantage. The possible advantage is that cancer of the breast, ovary, and lining of the womb are much less common among these people than in the West. This might be because the absence of ovarian hormones, with the ovaries themselves being switched off for years on end, makes cancer in the organs that normally respond to these hormones less likely. It has been suggested though that the difference might be accounted for by poor hospital facilities, with earlier death from other causes and no good record system.

The possible disadvantage that has been reported is premature ageing. Since the absence of ovulation in these women resembles that occurring after the menopause, it has been suggested that many of the changes that in Western women only occur after they have gone through the change of life begin to occur at a younger age in these women. This again is not easy to study and is more hypothesis than fact.

When Western women under laboratory conditions try and feed their babies regularly several things happen. It seems that ovarian function is switched off, with a gradual return as the frequency of feeding drops and the baby starts to take either solid food or a bottle. (It is perhaps worth noting that among the !Kung all children under the age of 12 months are fully breast-fed, while 90 per cent of those aged between one and two years are breast-fed. The percentage of babies dependent only on the breast for nourishment falls to only 75 per cent for those aged between two and three years.) In women who are studied carefully it seems that the first menstrual period after childbirth and breast-feeding comes before the first release of an egg, possibly because of the anti-fertility effect of the (by then decreasing) levels of prolactin on the ovary and the secretion of progesterone. This means that, in theory at least, women need not resume using contraception until they have had their first period after childbirth. In practice, possibly because most women do not feed with the same frequency as the !Kung do, pregnancies can occur. This possibly does not matter if the couple had been planning another baby anyway, but can be a source of distress if a baby was not wanted or was not wanted just at that time. Concern was once expressed that if a woman conceived whilst breast-feeding the obstetrician looking after her would be unable to estimate the length of her gestation accurately. Since the use of ultrasonic scanning became almost routine, and has been shown to be a much more sensitive indicator of gestational age than menstrual dates anyway, this worry has declined somewhat in importance.

One other point needs to be mentioned. In both men and women diseases leading to high levels of prolactin secretion are associated with decreased sexual feelings, with many men becoming impotent. Some women say that a similar thing happens to them when they breast-feed, and for them the superb contraceptive effect of breast-feeding occurs at a time when they do not feel much like sex anyway.

Other methods

In Chapter 2 we discussed some of the historical aspects of contraceptive use and it is worth emphasizing again the historical importance of natural methods. We know little about contraceptive practices of centuries ago, but we do know that the only methods available to ordinary people were these methods, with total abstinence and abortion being employed as well. It is however an historical fact that the birth rate has been declining in Western Europe, probably since the Industrial Revolution. Periods of recession—for instance the depression of the 1930s—were associated with marked declines. Most demographers think that these were too steep to be accounted for solely by illegal abortion and have suggested that perhaps coitus interruptus was responsible. It was probably not related to periodic abstinence because the method had not been studied as intensively then as now, and the Catholic church was not promoting it as widely as it is now.

Natural methods have many advantages over conventional methods. There are disadvantages, too, with perhaps their

Natural methods of family planning

biggest single advantage (their rapid reversibility) being closely linked with their biggest drawback. They need no medical supervision, but to be reliable perhaps need a lot of assistance from other people who, while not needing a lot of expensive training, do need a lot of enthusiasm and tact. For some couples the lack of absolute reliability, particularly for those who have completed their families, makes them want a more permanent, less intrusive means of avoiding pregnancy. Each year in the United Kingdom about 200 000 people make this decision and undergo voluntary sterilization. This topic will be covered in the next chapter.

10

Sterilization

Sterilization has one major difference from the other methods of contraception which we have discussed in this book. It is permanent, and in most cases, irreversible. Clearly this means that a lot more thought needs to go into the decision to use it. In this chapter we will discuss what sterilization involves, who is likely to find it a suitable method, and what can be done if it does turn out to be a mistake.

Before a man or woman actually has a sterilization the doctor involved will want to make sure that they have been properly counselled. This counselling just means a discussion between the doctor or nurse and the couple (or person) to discuss clearly what is involved. This is an important precaution, because many people may have mistaken ideas about the nature of sterilization and the benefits they might get from it.

Who should have a sterilization?

While the permanence of sterilization is its main advantage it is also the main drawback. This makes it important not to choose sterilization just because there are side-effects or difficulties with other methods. The person being sterilized must be in a situation where they are absolutely sure that they cannot think of any circumstances where they would wish to have a child. In practice, this means that most people requesting sterilization are in their late twenties or early thirties, have two or three children, and are relatively happily married. It is thought in fact that in some Western countries perhaps one-third of recently married couples will finally choose sterilization. It may well be equally suitable for a woman in her forties who, although unlikely to fall pregnant, is really worried about the possibility. At the other end of the scale, more and more women in Western society are making a conscious decision never to have children, and they may want to seek a sterilization at a much younger age. Another group of people who may wish to have a sterilization are those who know that their children would inherit a serious disease and so feel that they should not reproduce.

When a couple have decided that they do want a sterilization, there is then the question of which partner should be sterilized. This depends partly on their feelings when they know what male and female sterilization involves, but there may be other factors. If there is a large age gap between the two partners, it may be sensible for the elder to be sterilized, so that the younger could if necessary remarry and have children. Men often feel that as women have been through childbirth it should be men who should go through an operation for sterilization, especially since the operation is much less complicated for men.

What does sterilization involve?

The principle of sterilization is the same for both men and women. It is a small operation which aims to block the tubes carrying the sperms or eggs in order that fertilization can no longer take place. This is *all* either operation does. There is no effect on the individual's hormones or their general health, or sexual feelings (though it is important to note that if you are having sexual or marital difficulties with your partner before the operation, these are rarely made better by the operation and can be made worse). For the woman sterilization does not interfere with the womb or the ovaries, so periods continue as before, and the timing of menopause is not appreciably altered.

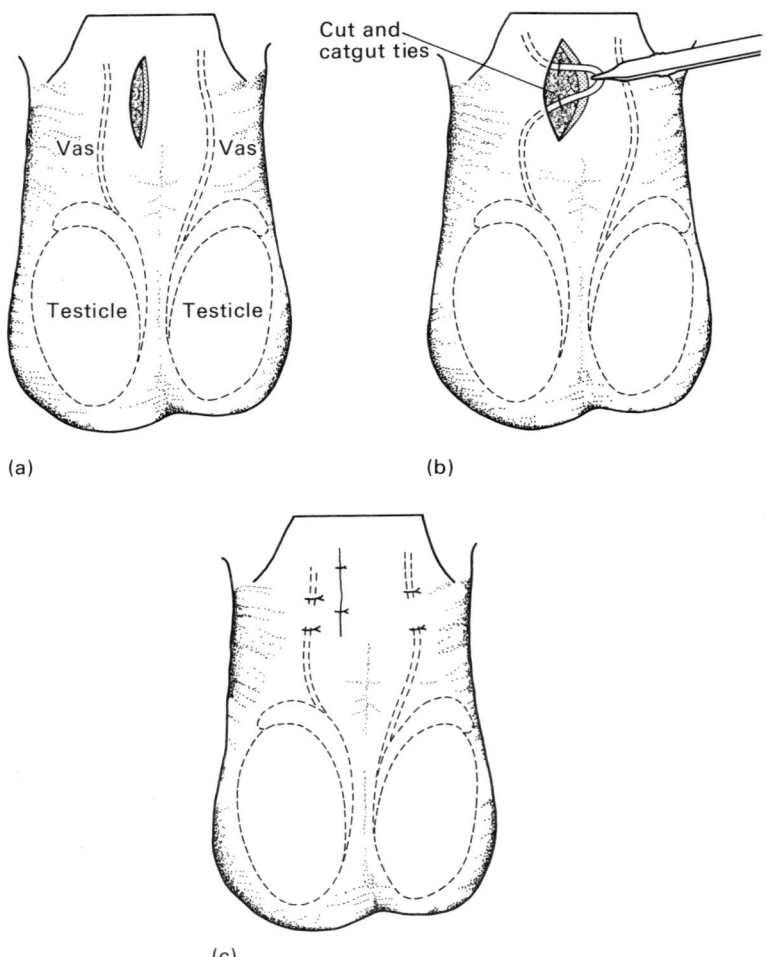

Fig 10. **Male sterilization. Stages of the vasectomy operation: (a) skin incision in scrotum; (b) identification of vas; (c) vasa cut and tied and skin incision sutured.** (From Foley, M. *Contraception,* Update Publications, London.)

Male sterilization: vasectomy

The word 'vasectomy' means cutting of the 'vas', and this, properly called the 'vas deferens', is the muscular tube which carries spermatozoa from the site of their production in the testes to the outside. Vasectomy is normally performed under a local anaesthetic, though a general anaesthetic can be used. A small injection is made into the skin of the scrotum just over the vas. This makes the skin numb so that a small cut can then be made in order to reach the tube, divide it, and tie the ends (Fig. 10). The same procedure is then repeated on the other side. Sometimes a single incision is made in the mid-line of the scrotum so that the end result is only one small cut which usually only requires one or two stitches. The operation normally takes 20 minutes or less and if you have it done under a local anaesthetic you will be able to leave the clinic straight away.

After the operation, you are advised to wear tight underpants or an athletic support (or jock-strap) day and night for the following couple of weeks. This is because there is always a little bruising around the site of the operation, and the skin around the testes is loose and elastic so that a very large bruise can build up unless continuous pressure is applied. This bruising and the formation of a big swelling, called a haematoma, is the commonest complication of a vasectomy, although it only happens to a minority of men. Fortunately, although it is uncomfortable while it lasts, it usually settles down fairly quickly. The other useful thing to do is to bath regularly with a little salt added to the water. This helps to keep the cuts clean while they are healing. In fact, infection usually occurs together with bruising so that keeping the bruising to a minimum will also prevent infection.

The other important point about a vasectomy involves the question of how quickly it will work. There are many millions of sperms 'down-stream' of the point where the vas is blocked, and so this means that you are still fertile for some weeks after the operation. How long you remain fertile depends very much on how often you ejaculate. Most clinics usually suggest that a sample of semen produced by masturbation should be brought to the clinic at three months and a further sample at four months. If no sperms can be found in either of these samples then the operation has been successful and you are no longer fertile. In practice, spermatozoa are usually cleared from the body a lot sooner, and after 20 ejaculations there are unlikely to be significant numbers left. Obviously it is important to continue using contraception until the semen has been carefully checked.

Many people wonder what happens to the sperms (or after female sterilization, the eggs) when the tubes have been blocked. These are still produced as usual, but when they are not used the body deals with them in the same way as any other unwanted cells. They are carried away and broken down in order to be used for new cells. There is no great 'sperm mountain' developing inside the body!

What other problems may arise?

We have already mentioned the immediate complications of bruising and infection. Like any operation, vasectomy may fail. This may be because the cut ends of the vas rejoin during the healing process, or even years later, or rarely, it may be because the man had a third (or even a fourth!) vas deferens. This makes it even more important to have the semen checks we described. If the vasectomy has not worked then it is usual for a surgeon to explore the vas deferens under a general anaesthetic.

Another but unusual complication of vasectomy is a harmless condition called sperm granuloma, which is a hard lump which forms at the cut end of the vas deferens. In some men this is just a small bump which can be felt in the scrotum, but in others it can become bigger and need removing.

The other worry which has been expressed in recent years is the possibility that vasectomy might have a more general effect on a man's health. Some experiments done on monkeys suggested that there was an increased incidence of problems with the circulation, particularly the clogging up of the blood-vessels and conditions such as heart attacks. It seems however that this can be applied only to the animals on which the research was being carried out, and a number of big studies looking at thousands of men after vasectomy suggest that there is no difference between their health and that of the rest of the population. Other studies have also shown men generally to be well pleased with the results of the operation.

Female sterilization

The principle of female sterilization is to block each of the Fallopian tubes which carry eggs from the ovaries to the womb. These tubes are inside the abdomen and we do not yet have a reliable technique for blocking them without a small operation. This means that the procedure involves either a laparotomy, a laparoscopy, or a culdotomy. A laparotomy involves a small incision in the abdomen, usually about three to four inches long and going across the bottom of the abdominal wall. There is also a version of this called a 'mini-laparotomy' which is the same in principle but involves a smaller cut. A laparoscopy is a more modern technique which is now very widely used. It involves inserting a telescope-like instrument (the laparoscope) into the abdomen through a small cut underneath or through the navel. We will be talking more about this later in the chapter. Culdotomy means entering the abdominal cavity through a cut in the vagina. This is a popular way of reaching the tubes for sterilization in some countries, but is rarely used in the West. Some individual surgeons in countries like Bangla Desh have done many thousands of these operations with very few problems. The surgeon doing the sterilization procedure will choose the best method for any particular women, after considering not only his personal skills but also the circumstances of the woman to be operated on.

Contraction:

Laprotomy

As the aim of sterilization is to block the tubes effectively, while causing them the least damage, a number of different techniques have been evolved. The simplest of these entails picking up a loop of Fallopian tube and tying a stitch around it, before cutting out a segment. The disadvantage of this is that the ends of the canal within the tube may find one another and rejoin. There are a number of ways of avoiding this which vary from burying one end of the tube in the wall of the womb, or one of its supporting ligaments, to fixing the ends in such a position that they cannot reach one another. These methods of laparotomy sterilization are all quite simple and usually take 10 to 20 minutes when performed under a general anaesthetic. A local anaesthetic can be used if there is some reason for avoiding a full anaesthetic, but this is not widely done. In some centres spinal or epidural anaesthetic is used. This involves injecting local anaesthetic drugs into, or around, the spine.

Laparoscopy

However, these techniques have largely given way to the use of the laparoscope. This instrument is like a narrow telescope. The operation is normally performed under a general anaesthetic, though a local anaesthetic may be used. Gas is inserted into the abdomen in order to allow the internal organs to separate and make room for the instrument. A small cut is made in or through the navel and the laparoscope is introduced to give a view of the womb, ovaries, and Fallopian tubes. Some laparoscopes have other attachments added to them. Most people make a second, small cut (less than a centimetre long) in the lower abdomen. Through this a second instrument can be inserted and the tube blocked by this under direct vision from the laparoscope.

There are a number of ways of blocking the tube with this technique. The original method was 'diathermy coagula-

128

tion', where an electrical current was passed through the tube, heating a section of it to the point where it was destroyed. This tends to leave only a small portion of the tube intact, and the amount of heat required sometimes damaged other organs in the pelvis. Because we occasionally try to reverse sterilizations, other less damaging techniques have been introduced. These take the form of clips or small silicone-plastic rings which can be placed over the tube.

The whole operation takes about 15 to 20 minutes and the patient recovers more quickly than from a laparotomy. However it is not always technically possible to insert the laparoscope, and certainly anyone who is very overweight, or who has scars on the abdominal wall from previous operations, needs to be aware that it may not be possible to use this technique.

Following sterilization by the laparoscopic method, most women are well enough to go home the same day, though a lot of hospitals suggest that they stay overnight. The main discomfort during the 24 hours afterwards is not always in the abdomen. The gas which we referred to earlier irritates the bottom of the diaphragm and causes a phenomenon called referred pain, which means that the main discomfort may be felt in the shoulder tip. If clips or rings have been put on the tubes, the muscle of the tubes will often go into spasm at first and this may give some crampy pain in the lower abdomen. The operation leaves two small scars, one at the site of entry of each instrument, but these soon fade and are not really noticeable.

As with vasectomy, female sterilization can fail, though women are much less likely to fall pregnant after a sterilization than if they were to stay on the pill for the rest of their lives. While most failures will result from the ends of the tubes having rejoined, there are also rarely technical errors when using the laparoscopic method. This is because the laparoscope only gives a narrow field of view and in someone where previous disease has made the tubes hard to see, it is possible for the clip or ring to be put on the wrong place. Unfortunately, when female sterilizations fail there is an increased chance of the resulting pregnancy remaining in the tube. This is of course because the tube has been deliberately blocked, and if it becomes partly unblocked then the fertilized egg may have difficulty travelling down into the womb.

What other problems may arise?

Many women are worried about the possible effect of sterilization on their periods or on their production of hormones. Modern techniques of sterilization aim to block the Fallopian tube with the minimum effect on surrounding structures, and hormone levels should not normally be altered. It is often claimed that about a quarter of all women having sterilizations complain that their periods become heavier after the operation. There may be a number of reasons for this, but one is certainly that many women will have been having light 'periods' on the pill until the time of the operation, and when they come off the pill they revert to normal, somewhat heavier patterns of bleeding. Another possibility may be that a period seems heavier when it no longer serves the purpose of reassuring you that you are not pregnant. Certainly the only study which has actually measured the amount of blood lost at each period before and after sterilization did not show any difference.

It is also often said that women having a sterilization later end up having a hysterectomy. It is important to remember that very many women in their late thirties and early forties have a hysterectomy in order to cure period problems. So since both sterilizations and hysterectomies are very common operations many women will have both. This does not mean that there is any direct connection, of course, and there has been no definite proof of one yet.

Sterilization

When should sterilization be done?

As we have said, sterilization should really only be considered when the couple (or individual, if there is no permanent partner involved) are absolutely certain that they will not want another child. 'Absolutely certain' tends to be a relative term, and there must be few people who have not changed their minds about something they were once very sure of. There are particular times when people are more likely to make a decision which they later regret. We would not recommend anyone to consider sterilization immediately after a child is born. The few days after the birth of a baby used to be a popular time for sterilization for women, because it avoided a return to hospital at a later date when there might be no-one to look after the children. Studies have been made of women some years after sterilization, and it seems that those who had their operation immediately after the birth of a baby are more likely to regret this later. This may be partly because feelings change during a pregnancy, but also the first few days of life are among the most dangerous for a baby, and there is a lot to be said for waiting a few weeks to see that the latest child is well.

We would give the same advice about sterilization after termination of pregnancy. It is very tempting when someone feels that her family is complete and is requesting an abortion to think of having a sterilization at the same time, and take away the worries of a further unwanted pregnancy. However, combining abortion with sterilization does increase the risks of the operation as well as being an action which may be regretted later.

It is worth repeating briefly the main factors which are associated with regretting the decision to have a sterilization. The most obvious of these is age. Studies show that many people having a sterilization under the age of 25 are unhappy about this later, though this does not necessarily mean of course that they want the sterilization reversed.

Contraception: the facts

Many couples who are experiencing difficulties with their marriage or with the sexual side of their relationship may feel that a sterilization may help 'to save the marriage'. Unfortunately, this often does not seem to be the case, and anyone whose relationship either is, or has recently been, breaking up should avoid having a sterilization at that time. The other group which we have mentioned are those who have just completed a pregnancy. It is almost certainly worth waiting at least six weeks after a pregnancy before either partner has a sterilization. One point to think about is that while it is one thing not to want a pregnancy, it is another to know that you are no longer capable of having one.

Reversal of sterilization

What can be done if someone has had a sterilization and later wants it reversed? As we have said, sterilization should be looked on as an irreversible operation, but it is sometimes possible to reverse it successfully. This depends partly on the technique which has been used for the operation.

Reversal in men

Reversal of vasectomy involves an operation in which the ends of the vas are found, opened up, and then joined together with very fine stitches. This is a skilled operation and the few surgeons who perform this tend to have fairly long waiting lists. Unfortunately, while it is possible to rejoin the ends of the tube, this does not always make a man fertile again. Although the operation enables the man's sperms to travel down the vas deferens his immune system might have started producing antibodies against his sperms. It is unclear why this happens, but it means in effect that the man attacks his own sperm as they are produced, and these antibody covered sperm are not as good as they ought to be at swimming through his partner's cervical mucus and fertilizing her eggs.

Sterilization

Reversal in women

Reversal of sterilization in women is much more dependent on the technique used originally. In order to have a reasonable chance of successfully rejoining the tube, at least three centimetres of the tube (about one-third) should be remaining. Diathermy sterilization which we mentioned earlier in the chapter, if done vigorously, destroys too much of the tube to allow reversal. Some surgeons also perform sterilization by removing a substantial part of the tube. The rings or clips cause the least damage to the tube and give the best chance for reversal. Reversal is still not an easy operation, partly because the Fallopian tube is not shaped like a pipe. It is in fact much wider at its outer end than at the end nearest the womb, and the result of removing or damaging the middle section of the tube may be that the surgeon then has to rejoin two ends of tube, one of which may be several times the diameter of the other. This operation can be done using the naked eye, but the best results are obtained when the surgeon uses an operating microscope. Here the surgeon looks through something like a pair of binoculars at the Fallopian tubes and so is able to use instruments and stitches which are extremely small and delicate. Because this surgery is so highly skilled there are again only a small number of surgeons who are interested in reversal of sterilization, and their waiting lists tend to be long.

Before being put on the waiting list for this kind of surgery it is usual to suggest a laparoscopy first in order to look closely at the tubes and assess the chances of a successful reversal.

For many people reversal of sterilization is either not possible or the surgical attempt fails. If the couple still want to try and have children there are only two options left for them. If the man is still sterile, his partner can be inseminated with semen from another man. This is a fairly simple procedure known as artificial insemination with donor semen. It has been estimated that about 20 000 babies are born each year after this procedure throughout the world. While the vast majority of these result from infertile marriages, a growing proportion result from relationships where the male partner has had a vasectomy. Some of them have not managed to have their vasectomy reversed, while others have not wanted it reversed: the potential discomfort and the thought that they would have to worry about contraception again were far too much for them.

For women who have not managed to have their sterilizations reversed the outlook is not as good. In years to come, when the techniques of *in vitro* fertilization and embryo transfer (the 'test-tube baby') are better established, then this might be a better alternative, better even than surgical attempts at reversal. All of the centres doing this form of research say that a small proportion of the women involved have had sterilizations performed that they now regret; in years to come they might form the biggest group.

In summary, there is no doubt that sterilization provides a safe, simple and reliable way of ensuring that you do not have any further children. For most people it is irreversible, and so a lot of thought should be given to choosing this method of contraception.

11

Abortion

This chapter differs from the others in that it is not truly about contraception. Abortion is the ending of a pregnancy, usually in its early stages, rather than its prevention. This is always second best to effective contraception, but all over the world abortion is one of the ways of dealing with unwanted pregnancies. There are about 30 million abortions performed every year, and at least half of these are illegal. In most countries making laws against abortion has only resulted in their continuing to be carried out, but under secret and often less safe circumstances.

Since good methods of contraception are readily available in Western society, why are there still so many unwanted pregnancies? One obvious reason is that many people still do not use contraception regularly. At least half of all young people starting their first sexual relationship use no contraception. Birth control can be an embarrassing subject to try and talk about with your partner at this stage especially when you are getting carried away by your feelings. Even among those using contraception reliably there will still be unwanted pregnancies due to failures of the method. Failure rates of modern methods may vary from less than one to five or more per cent, but these are risks per year and with a large sexually active population there will always be some pregnancies, even after many years of successful use. There are also those couples in whom a change of circumstances means that a pregnancy which would have been acceptable becomes unwanted during the few weeks after conception.

In recent years a further group of women requesting abortion has appeared. Doctors are getting progressively better at developing tests which will determine in the first part of the pregnancy whether the fetus is growing into a normal baby. Certain types of disability, such as chromo-some abnormalities, e.g. Down's syndrome (mongolism) and spina bifida can be detected fairly accurately. This has led to a group of women who may request abortion near the end of the first half of their pregnancy, after an abnormality has been discovered.

It is not our intention in this chapter to discuss moral views about abortion in detail. Here we discuss some of the facts about abortion which may help to make your own feelings clearer.

Abortion laws

As we have said, abortion is illegal in some countries of the world and restricted or governed by the law in some way in most other countries.

In the United Kingdom abortion is only legal if the 1967 Abortion Act is complied with. This Act requires two doctors to sign a form. In order to sign this they must form the opinion, in good faith, that one of four sets of circumstances apply. These are:

1. The continuance of the pregnancy would involve risk to the life of the pregnant woman greater than if the pregnancy were terminated.
2. The continuance of the pregnancy would involve risk of injury to the physical or mental health of the pregnant woman greater than if the pregnancy were terminated.
3. The continuance of the pregnancy would involve risk of injury to the physical or mental health of the existing child(ren) of the family of the pregnant woman greater than if the pregnancy were terminated.
4. There is substantial risk that if the child were born it would suffer from such physical or mental abnormalities as to be seriously handicapped.

The interpretation of this is left very much to the doctor so there are many different interpretations of what constitutes reasonable grounds for signing this form. Many doctors believe that there is reasonable evidence that it is damaging to a woman's psychological health to continue with a pregnancy that she does not want to keep, and so for them the majority of women who make a definite decision to request abortion have grounds for this.

Legally abortion can be carried out in the United Kingdom up to the 28th week of pregnancy, but this law has been outdated by improvements in the care of very premature babies. A pregnancy which ends in the 28th week can now often produce a baby who would survive and so, except in unusual circumstances, it is very rare to perform abortion after the 20th week of pregnancy.

The situation in the United States of America is very different. In the late 1960s and early 1970s many states began to liberalize their laws, but this procedure was overtaken in 1973 by the Supreme Court ruling that the laws as they then stood were unconstitutional. The Supreme Court ruled strongly in favour of the rights of the pregnant woman, and argued that the abortion decision should be one between the woman and her doctor.

This decision was based partly on the medical practices that had been in force at the time that the Constitution and Bill of Rights had been enacted, and partly on the definition of 'persons' who were allowed to have 'constitutional rights'. Abortion had been freely available in the early days of American society, and the founding fathers had made it clear that a fetus did not count as a person.

The judgement concluded that:

it is thus apparent that at common law, at the time of the adoption of our Constitution, throughout the major portion of the nineteenth century, abortion was viewed with less disfavour than under most American statutes currently in effect. Phrasing it another way, a woman enjoyed a substantially broader right to terminate a pregnancy than she does in most states today. At least with respect to the early stage of pregnancy, and very possibly without such a limitation, the opportunity to make this choice was present in this country well into the nineteenth century.

137

The net result of this has been the availability of abortion on request throughout the whole of the United States. This has been accompanied by an increase in the safety of the procedure, as more women approach their doctors earlier for what has become an open, available procedure.

The laws regarding abortion in other countries vary widely. Abortion may be completely illegal. This is still true of some countries but in certain of these termination of pregnancy is allowed if it is necessary to save the woman's life. Other countries allow abortion on specified grounds, which may be purely medical, such as the risk to the life or health of the pregnant woman, or a risk of abnormality in the fetus. They may be social grounds such as allowing the abortion of a pregnancy which follows rape or incest, or socio-medical grounds which usually allow a fairly wide degree of interpretation. There are also 20 countries where abortion is available to women on request without needing to meet any of these preconditions. However, even in these countries there are usually some limitations regarding either the woman's age, or the length of the pregnancy prior to termination. In Sweden women are entitled to abortion as a right in the first third of pregnancy, and in theory a doctor could go to prison if he refused one.

What does an abortion involve?

There are many ways of producing an abortion, and some of the simpler ways have been known to man for centuries. Research from the United States and Britain in the mid-nineteenth century suggests that abortion was very common then, with at least one-third of all women having one or more abortions. Most of these abortions were carried out by midwives and 'unqualified' people rather than doctors. The techniques were primitive compared to those available in the West today. However, in parts of the world outdated techniques are still used. In rural Thailand, for example, approximately 1 in 7 women has an illegal abortion each year, and the commonest technique is 'massage'. This involves very firm and painful massaging of the abdomen followed by direct squeezing of the womb. This painful and dangerous method often has to be repeated for a number of days before the fetus has been sufficiently crushed for it to be expelled by the womb. In other countries the use of various plant preparations either swallowed or injected into the womb are popular. In Western society abortion has been simplified into a number of safe and simple surgical methods. In this chapter we will concentrate on describing these methods.

The technique used to terminate a pregnancy depends largely on how far the pregnancy has progressed. The earlier in pregnancy that an abortion is carried out, the simpler and safer it is.

Methods up to 12 weeks

Menstrual extraction

The method which is used in the very early stages of pregnancy is often referred to as menstrual extraction or menstrual regulation, but this is probably something of a misnomer. If your period is about 10 to 14 days late and you think you are pregnant, the womb can be emptied by passing a fine plastic tube into it. This tube has an opening at its far end and the edge of the opening provides a surface suitable for scraping. The tube is attached to a vacuum-filled syringe and the combination of suction and scraping empties the womb. The advantage of this was originally thought to be that at this early stage of the pregnancy a very fine tube could be inserted and it would not be necessary to stretch up the entrance to the womb. This in turn would mean that a general anaesthetic was not required. In fact the actual process of emptying the womb causes quite a lot of discomfort, and in most places this particular method has been dropped.

D and C

The majority of women request abortion between 8 and 12 weeks after their last period. At this stage there are two commonly used techniques. The first is the well-known 'D and C' (dilatation and curettage). This is a procedure which is often performed under a general anaesthetic, though it can be equally well done with a local anaesthetic (a series of injections similar to those that a dentist uses). It involves stretching open (dilating) the entrance to the womb until an instrument can be inserted which will scrape (curette) the lining to remove the whole of the pregnancy. This technique is still very popular, but it has been improved by something called vacuum aspiration.

Vacuum aspiration

Vacuum aspiration involves a dilatation of the entrance to the womb very similar to that used in a D and C. However, instead of inserting a curette the doctor then inserts a metal or plastic tube similar to a larger version of that used for menstrual extraction. This is then attached to a suction pump and the contents of the womb are sucked out. These contents are then checked in order to make sure that the whole of the pregnancy has been removed.

Both D and C and vacuum aspiration have a number of advantages. They can be performed in 5 to 10 minutes under a general anaesthetic, and when you wake up it is all over. These are very safe procedures; in fact the risks involved in an abortion by one of these methods is less than the risks involved in continuing with the pregnancy. They also have the advantage that they do not normally cause any damage to the womb, and the amount of blood lost during the operation is very small. When you wake up from this sort of operation you will usually be bleeding less than you would during a normal period and you will have only a slight ache at the bottom of your abdomen.

The amount of stretching of the cervix which is required depends on how many weeks pregnant you are, and for this reason these techniques are only practical until about the end of the first three months. After that the use of this technique becomes less safe so in the second three months of pregnancy other methods are used.

Methods after 12 weeks

D and E

The most popular methods differ from one country to another. In some countries a technique called dilatation and evacuation (D and E) is commonly used. This can involve a general anaesthetic, which has the advantage that when you wake up the procedure is over. However, after 12 to 14 weeks it is not possible to suck the contents of the womb through a small tube and the insertion of a larger tube would be potentially damaging to the cervix. Because of this the cervix is stretched up to about the same amount as would be required for the vacuum aspiration technique and instruments are then inserted to crush the developing pregnancy and to bring it out from the womb in pieces. Although this is less safe than an abortion in the first three months of pregnancy, it is still a very safe technique to use from 12 to 18 weeks gestation. It has the advantage of being completed under a general anaesthetic, but it is not a pleasant operation for the medical or nursing staff involved.

For this reason a number of other techniques have evolved. These all depend on the use of some type of medicine which will cause the womb to start contracting, making the woman miscarry.

Intra-amniotic and extra-amniotic methods

One such technique is the intra-amniotic method. This involves using a local anaesthetic injected into the skin of the abdomen just above the womb. A needle is then inserted into the fluid around the developing pregnancy, and after drawing some of this fluid off, one or more of a number of drugs are injected into the space. Some of these drugs are concentrated solutions of salt or urea, while others, which may be used on their own or in conjunction with the salt solutions, are derivatives of the natural body hormone prostaglandin.

An alternative method of getting medicines into the womb is by the extra-amniotic route. This involves passing a flexible rubber tube through the entrance to the womb, a procedure which is very easy with a soft, pregnant cervix. Drugs can then be injected either continuously or at intervals through this tube in order to start the womb contracting. The commonest drugs given in this way are prostaglandins. Prostaglandins are a family of substances which occur naturally in the body. Two of them in particular have been found to cause contractions of the womb. They are often used to start labour in full-term pregnancies. When they are injected either directly into the womb or into the bloodstream in early pregnancy, they tend to produce abortion. This is a very safe technique, but there are a number of disadvantages.

Disadvantages. First, the side-effects of the prostaglandins are sickness and diarrhoea, and quite a lot of women receiving prostaglandins will experience this. Secondly, these medicines are inserted while you are awake and you then have to wait, often for some hours, before the womb starts to contract. You then have to go through the process of a miscarriage and if this is in the fourth or fifth month of pregnancy then it can be very distressing as well as uncomfortable. The other common problem is that at this stage of pregnancy the miscarriage will expel the growing fetus, but the developing afterbirth might be retained. This means that even after going through this process you may still need a general anaesthetic in order to remove the afterbirth. This method then, although very safe, is more traumatic for the woman involved.

Hysterotomy

In the past two other techniques have been used for abortion and these are still quite common in some parts of the world. One is hysterotomy, which involves a general anaesthetic and a major operation, in which the surgeon performs something like a Caesarean section by opening the womb and shelling out the contents. This can only be used for abortions relatively late in pregnancy and it is less popular nowadays.

Hysterectomy

For the woman who has completed her family surgeons sometimes suggest a hysterectomy termination. This involves terminating the pregnancy by removing the womb with its contents. Unless there are other medical conditions which make this a good idea, most doctors would feel that this is an unnecessary and relatively dangerous way of terminating a pregnancy.

In summary then—abortion during the second three months is technically possible. Up to 15 or 16 weeks of pregnancy it still remains safer than continuing with the pregnancy and giving birth. However, late abortions are not without their hazards and they tend to be much more distressing for both the women involved and the people taking care of them. It is partly for this reason that many countries allow abortion on request up to 12 weeks of pregnancy, but apply some restrictions after that. It is an unfortunate fact that the very people who come for a late abortion tend to be among those who are likely to be most distressed by the abortion, and they are also the people for whom it may be necessary to perform it by the most distressing technique. Among these are young girls who have not realized, or who have been scared to admit, that they are pregnant; older women who wanted the pregnancy but have discovered that it is not developing normally; and those whose circumstances have changed since they first fell pregnant.

Consequences of abortion

There has been a lot of often very emotional discussion and an equally large amount of careful scientific research about the possible consequences of abortion. Many of us, perhaps partly because of our doubts about the morality of abortion, have subconscious fears that there may be some 'punishment' in the form of illness or infertility which may stem from having one. This idea has been carried so far that in parts of the United States women have been asked to sign consent forms for abortion which clearly describe a number of disastrous consequences. However, there is no scientific support for this. Less than 1 per cent of all women having abortion have any problems at the time of abortion, and the earlier that they have the operation the less likely they are to have any problems (at least after seven weeks of pregnancy). It is perhaps important to emphasize that delay in seeking abortion does considerably increase the risks, and though these remain small this means that any woman who is sure that she wants termination of pregnancy should request this as early as possible and not be in any way deterred by her physician. It is known that one of the main causes of delay in receiving abortion is the tendency of many doctors to make people wait.

In the past people have been concerned about unfounded beliefs regarding the long-term complications of abortion. However, the truth remains that abortion is something which is becoming increasingly safer in our society, and which up to the 15th week of pregnancy is safer than childbirth. The chances of serious complications at the time of operation are less than those that are involved in having

144

your tonsils removed, while there is no firm evidence about any long-term effects of abortion on fertility or general health.

How do you decide whether to have an abortion?

Probably at least half of all pregnancies in Western society are unplanned. By no means all of these are unwelcome. However, the first response of many women to discovering that they are pregnant is one of panic and despair. It is only too easy under these circumstances to feel that an abortion will offer a magic solution to the crisis. This means that while for many women the decision to terminate the pregnancy will be unequivocal, many more will need some form of counselling. The object of counselling is for the counsellor (doctor, nurse, or friend) to share with the woman the problems associated with being pregnant. It is important, if only for one's future peace of mind, to think seriously about all the possible options. Even though the pregnancy may be unwanted it may be possible to come to terms with this and to have and keep the baby. Very often for some women, particularly the younger woman, continuing with the pregnancy and then offering the baby for adoption may be preferable to an abortion, particularly to the woman who has any moral objections to abortion. Either of these courses of action may be difficult and one of the aims of the counsellor is to provide continuing support in these situations.

First, it is important to explore what the pregnancy means to you. How do you feel about the relationship within which it was conceived? How do you feel about the idea of destroying that pregnancy? Are there are practical alternatives, or does it seem inevitable to you that you must have an abortion? Most people in this situation find that they are feeling rather ambivalent; that is to say that although they may have logical reasons for choosing one particular option, they may find that they have feelings which are pulling them in both directions. When this is so there are bound to be some negative feelings afterwards whatever decision you make, and so it is not surprising that some women feel unhappy either after an abortion or after a decision to continue with an unwanted pregnancy. It is important to discuss these feelings with those closest to you, but it is also often helpful to get an outsider, such as one may find at a pregnancy counselling clinic, who will be concerned about your feelings but will not be directly involved in the way that families and partners are. Such a counsellor may also be able to help you deal with the feelings that you may still have some months afterwards.

Contraception

We have already said that abortion must always come a very poor second to effective contraception. Within three weeks of having an abortion, over one-third of all women start to release eggs from their ovaries again, and within six weeks the proportion has risen to 4 out of 5. This does mean that contraception needs to be used as soon as love-making is resumed after an abortion, and this is a very important factor about which to make a decision before having an abortion. Which method you choose depends on the sort of factors that we have described in other chapters; the only advice which we would give is that it is not a wise time to have a sterilization. Sterilization increases the risks of abortion and you are much more likely to regret that you had this done if you combine the two operations.

Summary

In this chapter we have outlined a little about the techniques of abortion, its advantages and disadvantages, and the legal regulations which surround it. Many of us would feel much happier if there were simpler and still safer techniques which could be used by the woman herself in order that she could make a more truly independent decision. This is an area which is likely to change a lot over the next few years and we discuss this a little more in Chapter 12.

12

Contraceptives of the future

In the early 1970s a chapter on contraceptives of the future would have been full of exciting ideas, the products of which seemed to be just around the corner. Large sums of money were being put into contraceptive research, both by individual governments and by international organizations. Unfortunately the steam has now gone out of this movement, and most of the advances which we can expect in the near future are likely to be only minor improvements and variations on existing methods.

However, it is not only a lack of funding which is slowing the development of new contraceptive methods. Industrialized countries have become progressively more cautious about allowing products onto the market before their safety has been fully tested, and organizations such as the Food and Drug Administration (FDA) in the United States and the Committee on the Safety of Medicines (CSM) in the United Kingdom now have very stringent requirements in terms of the knowledge which must be accumulated about a drug before it can be brought into widespread use. The result of this is that even if one of our readers invented the perfect contraceptive technique today, it would probably be 10 to 15 years before it arrived on the market.

Despite this rather pessimistic start, there are a number of minor changes to existing methods in the pipeline, as well as some completely new methods. Perhaps it is worth looking at current methods first.

Spermicides

Barrier techniques still remain the most popular method of contraception in many countries, and their use could be increased considerably if some of the problems were removed. Spermicides are now being made with a cherry flavour, to counteract one of their main drawbacks for some users—their unpleasant taste. A new spermicide that works by stopping sperms from swimming is the blood-pressure lowering drug propranolol. Tablets of this drug put into the vagina seem to prevent pregnancy nearly all the time.

The condom

Condoms have already been improved considerably over the years, and it seems that acceptability is the main problem in their use rather than their efficiency. Coloured and textured sheaths are much more widely available now than they were ten years ago.

The diaphragm

The diaphragm on the other hand provides an area for research where many of the most basic questions are still unanswered. It has always been assumed that the spermicidal cream which is applied to the cap is an essential part of the method. People talk of the cap just being there to hold the spermicide in the right place. However, it is not at all certain whether this is true, and this argument applies even more in the case of the cervical cap or vimule. Current technology makes it possible to produce tailor-made caps which are made from a material which can be applied to the cervix and which will then set quickly, fitting exactly the contours of the neck of the womb in the particular woman who will be wearing it. It may be with these that the spermicide will not be necessary. A further sophistication of the cervical cap is one model which has a trap door, or valve, in it which will allow the menstrual fluid to come away so that the cap may be left in place continuously. Early trials have not shown much promise, but work continues.

Sponges

One of the earliest methods of contraception was to insert a sponge soaked in vinegar or lemon juice into the vagina. Interestingly this idea has now come full circle and synthetic sponges impregnated with spermicides are being tried out. These sponges become soft and release their spermicides in response to the natural moisture of the vagina. Some of these sponges can be reused, while others are disposable. One of them, at present being tried out in Arizona, looks rather like a powder puff.

The IUCD

The intrauterine contraceptive device has seen gradual improvements rather than any great leaps forward. The recent incorporation of a silver core into the copper wire will lead to a longer life for each device, and the shape is gradually being improved so that IUCDs will tend to stay at the top of the cavity of the womb. Hormone-containing coils have been tried in the past, and although these are not currently popular in the United Kingdom, they have by no means been discontinued. Research is going on at the moment to decide which hormones work best and in what dose.

The pill

The pill has really been perfected so much in recent years that it seems unlikely that there will be any great new improvement there. It seems that pills with hormone dosages that change during the cycle will probably be more popular, and the drug companies are certainly working hard to produce pills which will have an even smaller effect on the body. One other possibility with the pill is give the hormones which it contains by another route, and a number of techniques for this are being examined. There are some scientists who suggest the ordinary pill is just as effective and even safer when inserted into the vagina.

Vaginal rings

In some countries vaginal rings are being tested. These are circular silastic rings which the woman can fit into her vagina and which contain within them the same chemicals as the pill. These hormones slowly leak out through the plastic and are absorbed through the vagina. It certainly saves remembering to take anything, but one of the snags seems to be that many women get a slightly increased vaginal discharge with this. Like the pill, it can be used either for three weeks out of four, or continuously.

Implantation of hormone pellets into the fat under the skin also gives a potential way of providing something like the pill without having to swallow it. This, and other routes of administration, like nasal sprays, have been tried out in the hope that there might be some way of getting the hormones into the body to have a full contraceptive effect while reducing the side-effects still further. This does not seem to be very successful so far but people are still trying.

Nasal sprays

One development that might be in wider use before the end of the decade depends on interference with the hormones that control ovulation, but in a different fashion to the way the pill works. We mentioned in the first chapter that ovulation is under the control of the pituitary, and this in turn is controlled by the hypothalamus. The hypothalamus controls the pituitary by the release of small, regular pulses of gonadotrophin release hormone, or GnRH. The pituitary is very sensitive to this hormone, and if it is saturated with lots of it, or similar molecules that it cannot break down easily, it will cease to function. This will stop the production of the gonadotrophins, FSH and LH, and ovulation will not occur.

Unfortunately, GnRH is a protein, and so cannot be given by mouth. (If it is the gut digests it just as it would any other protein, and so its action is lost.) To prevent women from having to inject themselves every day the drug is put into an aerosol spray, and breathed in as a fine mist through the nose. Very tiny quantities of the hormone are absorbed from the lining of the nose, and these tiny quantities are enough to prevent ovulation. Early reports from Scotland and Sweden are that it is safe, effective, and easy to use. The women who have used it have been happy with it and have suffered no ill effects. The biggest problem has been cost—at the moment it costs about £200 for one month's treatment. It will certainly become cheaper when genetic engineering techniques allow economical production of large quantities of protein hormones, but at the moment it is too expensive to be anything other than an interesting research tool. Molecules that are similar in shape to GnRH might work in a similar fashion, and be cheaper. All of these drugs might only be needed for a few days in each month, which will make them cheaper and easier.

Sterilization

In sterilization the main object is to make the operation simpler, and yet at the same time more reversible.

Male sterilization

With vasectomy some workers have developed a kind of 'tap'. This can be inserted into the vas deferens and left in the off position while a very simple operation can then be done to turn the flow of sperms back on. We have not yet got as far as the point where you can control your own tap!

Contraceptives of the future

Female sterilization

In female sterilization, besides improving the clips which we discussed in Chapter 10, people are also looking for different routes for blocking the tubes. Scientists have experimented with types of 'super glue', trying to squirt this into the tubes from below and block them, but this has been technically somewhat difficult. Others have recently devised a small plastic tube which will fit within the Fallopian tube and block it. This can also be inserted through the uterine cavity using an instrument called the hysteroscope. This is rather like the laparoscope except that it gives a view of the inside of the womb, and using this it is possible to apply electrical current, or 'super glue', or nylon sheaths, or caustic chemicals to the inside of the bottom end of the tube as it enters the cavity of the womb. All these techniques are still being developed and some seem to offer promise.

Abortion

In abortion there is still a need to develop techniques which can be administered by the woman herself, as this makes the abortion decision a social and legal decision rather than a medical issue. The hope here is the prostaglandin pessary. These pessaries are small, bullet-shaped objects containing a synthetic version of the naturally occurring chemicals, prostaglandins, which were mentioned in the last chapter. The ideal which is being aimed for here is a substance which can be put into the vagina very early in pregnancy to produce an abortion without side-effects or the need for admission to hospital.

The male pill

We could hardly complete a book on contraception without talking about the male pill, although sadly there is not a lot to say about it. There would obviously be advantages of having a pill which could be taken by men, but there are some practical problems. The first of these is that almost any chemical which reduces sperm production also reduces sexual interest—not quite the way a contraceptive should work! The other problem is that the 'production line' which leads to fully formed sperm actually represents a process which is about 12 weeks long. This means that any male pill takes time to work, and equally, time to wear off.

Initially male and female sex hormones were tried as male pills, but more recently other techniques have been tried. It was found in China that men living in some areas had a naturally low fertility, and this was finally traced to an ingredient in the cotton-seed oil which they used for cooking. An extract of this, now called gossypol, is being tested extensively in China. Early trials were encouraging, although there were very high rates of side-effects. The most serious side-effect was muscular weakness produced by lowering the body's reserves of potassium. Some scientists think that very low concentrations of gossypol are effective at blocking the power of sperms to fertilize eggs. The concentrations of the drug are much lower than have been tried in the past, and it may be possible for side-effects to be avoided by giving very low doses. There has even been a suggestion that gossypol can be used as a spermicide, thus putting the contraceptive burden back on women! On the other side of the world in Latin America, other plant extracts are being tested both as a male contraceptive pill and for their effect in producing abortions.

Vaccines

One of the most attractive ideas which has appeared in contraception is the thought of 'immunizing' people against pregnancy. This would be a reversible method which would allow people to have an injection rendering them infertile for a given period of time. These methods, unfortunately,

Contraceptives of the future

have not really come to fruition—there are many technical reasons for this.

Scientists trying to prepare a contraceptive vaccine have worked along three main lines. They have tried to prepare vaccines against spermatozoa, for use by either men or women, or vaccines against the outer coverings of the egg, for use by women. The third track has been to prepare vaccines specifically against pregnancy, to try and make sure that any pregnancy that forms is rejected.

Contraceptive vaccines have been developed for many male animals. Some infertile men produce antibodies to their own spermatozoa, and they can impregnate their wives after the antibody levels have been lowered by means of steroid drugs. It is also known that men who have vasectomies often produce antibodies to spermatozoa, and that these antibodies may be responsible for the relatively low rates of success of reversal operations. Given these facts, it would seem that a male vaccine would be a potentially fruitful line of research.

Unfortunately this has not been the case. When animals are treated to make them infertile, they need an injection into the testis. It does not always work, and sometimes needs to be repeated. When it does work it is permanent, and sometimes it also leads to damage to the testis which reduces its ability to produce male hormones.

Antibodies to spermatozoa exist in women, but they are much harder to study. Medical folklore says that prostitutes are infertile because they are exposed to so many different types of semen that they eventually become immune to them all. Some careful studies have shown that many prostitutes do have high levels of antibodies to spermatozoa, while others have suggested that the incidence is just the same in virgins. Nobody has managed to produce a reliable antispermatozoa antibody for female animals yet.

Antibodies to the outer coverings of the egg are a much more promising field to investigate. Some infertile women do seem to have these antibodies in their blood, and in experimental animals it has been shown that these antibodies prevent spermatozoa from entering the egg. In years to come it might be possible to prepare a pure extract of the outer covering of the egg (the zona pellucida) and use this as the basis for a vaccine. The animal work suggests that booster injections would need to be given every year. This work is still decades away from being tried in humans, but since it would not interfere with hormones and ovulation it might be the basis for a good contraceptive.

Much more controversial is a 'pregnancy' vaccine. All early pregnancies produce a hormone called *H*uman *C*horionic *G*onadotrophin (HCG) that is essential for the maintenance of the pregnancy. It is a protein, and the antibody reaction to it is the basis for nearly all of the current pregnancy tests. In humans it does not seem to produce an immune response, but it does so when it is linked up with other molecules, like, for example, tetanus toxoid (the source for vaccines against tetanus). The combination of HCG and tetanus toxoid has been given to women, and has made them appear to be immune to HCG. For ethical reasons only women who had already been sterilized were involved, and so we do not know if it would have worked as a contraceptive for them.

The most controversial aspect about this line of research is the fact that women would be being immunized against one of the pregnancy hormones. While this would prevent pregnancy at such an early stage that it would probably never be noticed by the women, the widespread use of this vaccine would generate more concern than any other contraceptive measure.

Natural methods

Improvement of these methods will continue and one of the latest developments is the 'dipstick' urine test. At ovulation, the dipstick dipped in a urine sample changes colour, and combined with the dates of your periods, this information can be used to calculate the infertile 'safe time' for intercourse.

Conclusion

In our densely populated world, one new child is born every quarter of a second, and we can expect the world's population to double in the course of the next 40 years. The most important question is probably not whether we can develop new methods of contraception, but rather if we can get people to use the methods which are already in existence.

From this point of view we have seen some progress. Most countries in the world are beginning to assert some control over their population levels, and in the West surveys show people have an increased knowledge of contraceptive methods and of their availability. The use of reliable contraception, which was initially a middle-class prerogative, has gradually spread through the social classes. Doctors have finally been persuaded to become directly involved in giving contraceptive advice and to see this as part of their job; quite a contrast to their attitude only 50 years ago when they were actively fighting the spread of knowledge about birth control.

However, what we still do not have is equality of availability throughout the world of contraceptive methods, abortion and sterilization, and knowledge.

13

Where do I go from here?

So far in this book we have discussed most of the useful methods of contraception in some detail and given a pointer to future developments. By now you may be very clear about the method that suits you at this point in your life, but in this chapter we are going to look at the special problems of family planning for certain groups of women. Some of these women have medical conditions that mean that special care is needed, while others may need different methods at different stages in their lives.

The suggestions that we make in this chapter are not necessarily those that your own doctor or clinic would make, but they are an attempt to suggest what might be the 'best buy' for women in each group. Your own choice on contraception is a very individual matter, and you may or may not feel comfortable with the first medical advice you are offered. The last few pages of this book suggest alternative sources of family planning help.

Family planning needs throughout life are not constant. They will depend not only on how important it is to avoid pregnancy, but also on the changes in your own natural fertility and variations in the risk of the contraceptive method with age. We discussed in Chapter 2 how women are at their most fertile between the ages of 20 and 30, when some are building families and others careers. For those in the former an unplanned pregnancy is not necessarily a disaster, while for the latter a pregnancy could mean the end of their career. For some women an unplanned pregnancy means an early, safe, abortion and then resumption of normal life but, as we discussed in Chapter 11, the agonizing heart-searching that some women go through can be destructive to them, their careers, and their relationships,

Where do I go from here?

whether the end result is an abortion or not. People are now so sure that they can avoid an unwanted pregnancy that when one occurs they may find it harder to accept than they would have done a generation ago.

Sociologists divide women into three groups of contraceptive users: the delayers, the spacers, and the stoppers. The delayers are those women, usually young, who intend to become pregnant eventually but would none the less feel that it was a disaster if it came too soon. The spacers are those women who have had at least one child and would like another, but not yet; while the stoppers want no more pregnancies. There is also another group which is becoming gradually larger—the stoppers who have never started. While we have always accepted that no method of contraception can ever be absolutely effective, it is worth emphasizing that the same method of contraception has different failure rates in these different groups. This is why we have always quoted ranges for the effectiveness of different measures, and why we have said that bald figures on their own are not enough to help you make up your mind. Your age, your previous fertility, your need for contraception and the group which you fall into are all important. This book has provided the facts but the final decision must be yours. This decision may of course be influenced by your personal and religious beliefs.

Most religions have views on procreation and offer guidance to their believers about the acceptability of contraception. Bhuddism is probably the only major religion that does not have a history of encouraging its members to 'be fruitful and multiply'. Obviously these beliefs made sense in the past when the world's population was small and the strength of individual groups depended on their numbers. In the overcrowded and starving world of today most religions are prepared to allow much more individual freedom than they once did. In Western Europe most people make up their own minds on contraceptive use without referring to their religious leaders, but it is instructive to give an outline of the beliefs of various religions.

Christianity

Roman Catholicism is the most conservative of the major denominations of Christianity as far as birth control is concerned. Strangely, this approach, for which the church is now well known, has only been developed in recent years. Until the last century the church had not made any pronouncements on this matter. The changes that occurred were related to changing beliefs about the ensoulment of the fetus and these were confirmed in *Humanae Vitae* which Pope Paul VI offered as a papal encyclical in 1968.

A strong belief in the sanctity of human life has been extended to the point where any artificial prevention of pregnancy is considered a sin. Rather strangely, however, artificial altering of a couple's sexual behaviour is considered acceptable and the Catholic church has done a lot to promote improvements in methods for detecting ovulation to assist couples in deciding when to abstain from inter-course and for how long. It is perhaps interesting to note that despite the conservative advice which Catholics should follow there are no obvious differences in this country in their actual use of contraception when compared with non-Catholics.

Most other Christian denominations are willing to approve of any method of contraception which is mutually acceptable to both partners. Their views on abortion, however, tend to show much more variation, with most accepting its need, and sympathizing with the woman, though regretting its necessity.

On a global scale Christianity is a minority religion, and with our society containing an ever-increasing number of people of other faiths, some discussion of these other religious beliefs is essential. Some of these faiths are very loosely structured with no central body to pronounce on religious doctrine: an example is the Rastafarian cult among West Indian youths.

Judaism

Many of the beliefs in our society today have evolved from our Judaeo-Christian moral tradition and it is interesting to see what the current beliefs of Judaism are. Judaism, like Christianity, divides into a number of groups with different levels of conservatism. Their views on contraception arise from a conflict between those views expressed in the Bible encouraging breeding and their own liberal tradition of improving family life and education. In addition, there is a conflict between the orthodox population, who will tolerate no departure from Biblical teachings, and those with a more liberal attitude.

The more conservative belief sees reproduction as a religious duty, but does allow a man who has fathered a son and a daughter to use 'natural' family planning methods. The use of any physical impediment to prevent conception is expressly forbidden except for health reasons. It is not clear whether or not the pill counts as a physical impediment. Those who are more liberal now accept the use of contraception to delay families but not prevent them altogether.

Abortion is forbidden under orthodox law unless the mother's life is in grave danger. A recent Israeli government fell in association with a plan for abortion law reform that was blocked by one of the minority religious parties.

Islam

Islam grew out of the same Middle-Eastern deserts that spawned Judaism and Christianity. There was a need to increase the size of the faithful population in a society surrounded by hostile non-believers. There is also a fatalistic belief that does not contemplate interference with the will of Allah. The position of women in Islamic society which involves a measure of seclusion and restriction of their freedom tends to limit their acceptance of family planning. This is not helped by the requirement for women to keep themselves covered in front of men, and since most doctors are men this makes examination impossible. The need for a son to bury the father means that they will want keep on trying for a son even if the first few pregnancies produce only daughters.

Menstrual bleeding restrictions make it difficult to accept IUCDs or the progestogen-only pill. Restrictions on the preparation of food and the woman's sexual life whilst menstruating obviously mean that any method making the woman bleed for longer is unlikely to be acceptable. This restriction is common to Hindu women as well. While these taboos can be maintained in a society where women are surrounded by sisters and sisters-in-law to help with the cooking, this can be a potential source of friction for isolated immigrant families in foreign countries.

Hindu women share some of the menstrual taboos and have a similar belief in the importance of sons. The Aitareya Brahmana states that 'By means of a son have fathers passed over the deep darkness. The self is born from the self, the son is a ship, well-founded, to ferry over . . . a son is a light in the highest heaven'.

Common to many Eastern people is the belief that the right hand is clean and the left hand is dirty. The right hand is for holding the Koran or for eating, while the left is for handling dirty or contaminated things or wiping oneself. This makes the insertion of a diaphragm difficult since both hands are needed for this.

Bhuddism

Bhuddism tends to place much emphasis on the ethos of the 'middle way', and so takes a realistic approach to the need to

162

keep human population to a level that is appropriate to the available resources. There is also an emphasis on the concept of withdrawing from wordly pleasure with the celibate life being highly valued.

Women's attitudes to contraception are not only based on their religious views but also on their attitudes to sexuality and their own bodies. The decision to use any particular method of contraception depends also on their own physical health and their feelings about a future pregnancy. Age is important, not only for its influence on these attitudes but also for its effect on the risks and side-effects of different methods.

The under-16 age group

Young women under the age of 16 face several problems. Just at a time when they may be experimenting with a new and exciting kind of relationship they are faced with a choice between bravely approaching a doctor or facing talking openly with their partner about the problem of getting him to use a sheath. (Even this assumes that he knows where to get one if he is too young to go into a pub and use a slot machine.)

Going to a clinic may be made even more difficult for girls under 16 because of the attitude of our society to sex amongst boys and girls of this age. Legally sexual relations with a girl under the age of sixteen is labelled 'unlawful sexual intercourse', although interestingly enough it is only the boy who is guilty of committing an offence. Neither the girl nor the doctor who provides contraceptive help is breaking the law. A further problem is that family planning doctors and nurses may naturally suggest to the girl that she should discuss the matter with her parents. This often seems a very frightening thing to do at this age, though in practice when you have the courage to do it you often find that it works out better than you expected.

For the under-sixteens there has been quite a change in medical attitudes about the best methods to use in recent years. At one time doctors were reluctant to prescribe the pill to young girls who had only recently started having periods, or were still growing, because of the possible ill-effects from switching-off their hormone production. Now we realize that this carries no risk, while on the other hand we tend to be less enthusiastic about the IUCD. Although the coil has the advantage that it does not need to be remembered, and mother cannot find out about it, the risks of infection that we mentioned in Chapter 7 are worrying, particularly as these risks are high in this age group. Any method which interferes with the actual act of making love may not be very popular at a time when you are still learning how to do it. All-in-all, this makes the low-dosage pill the best method of contraception for young girls.

The over-35 age group

At the other end of reproductive life the pattern is different. Most women over the age of 35 have already tried many of the methods which appeal to them. In general they are not such a suitable group for the combined pill (see Chapter 3). On the other hand, the average woman in her late thirties probably only releases an egg from her ovaries one month in three. This reduces her chances of getting pregnant and in effect means that other contraceptive methods become more reliable, making the progestogen-only pill and the IUCD more suitable at this age. There is less risk of infection now, although many women begin to get heavier periods as they approach the menopause and this may be aggravated by the coil. Barrier contraception can be an extremely effective method for well motivated couples in this age group and, in purely statistical terms, the safest method of all (from the point of view of mortality among the women using it) is the diaphragm, backed up by early abortion for any failures which may occur. As periods become more irregular, one worrying feature that disturbs many women is the longer gaps between periods, which may make them worried about possible contraceptive failures.

More women at this age, whether they have had children or not, are turning to sterilization either for themselves or their partners.

As we have suggested, the same woman will usually need to use different methods of contraception at different stages of her reproductive career. For example, prior to the birth of the first child avoidance of a pregnancy may be very important. To avoid the disaster of an unplanned pregnancy an absolutely effective method is needed and this reassurance best comes from the pill.

After the birth of a child, and while waiting for another, effectiveness is not so important. It may not be the end of the world if a pregnancy comes after four instead of five years. Less effective methods that suit some women, such as the natural methods or the progestogen-only pill, may be more appropriate.

After the last child has been born, a high level of reliability is needed again. Eventually this may be provided by a fully reversible method of sterilization but until then not all couples would be willing to take such an irrevocable step. The birth of the last child does not usually coincide with the falling fertility of the 35-year old, and so for this group the pill often remains the 'best buy'.

The disabled

Contraception can be a fiddly thing at the best of times, even for the able-bodied. People who are limited in their freedom of movement may find some methods difficult. They may find a diaphragm difficult to use and the heavier periods that the IUCD produces more than they can cope with. The pill has the advantage of being the simplest method mechanically. There is the theoretical problem that if someone is relatively immobile the risks to the circulation may be greater but this is outweighed by the advantages.

The sheath can also be a problem if either partner has restricted movements. Men can find it a problem to put on while, if their partner is so restricted as to make intercourse difficult, the sheath can come off or be torn.

Many doctors stress the benefits of sexual activity in people with arthritis, and there have been several reports of pain relief lasting several hours after sex. When disability isolates people maintaining the intimate side of a relationship becomes even more important, and the physically disabled would be well advised to make sure they get the best possible advice on contraception.

Some disabled people feel they would be unable to cope with child-bearing and request sterilization at a much earlier stage in their relationships than others. We would of course support this, but the other side of the coin is that many people with a physical disability find child-rearing especially rewarding.

However, it is not only those with physical limitation of their movement who may have special requirements for contraception. A number of other life-long conditions require special consideration. We would like to illustrate this with two examples—diabetes and epilepsy.

Diabetics

Diabetic women often experience rather more difficulties with pregnancy than other women. This is partly because of the difficulties in controlling the levels of sugar in their blood that may occur in pregnancy, and partly because some of the complications of pregnancy seem to happen more often to diabetic women. It is extremely important that a diabetic woman only has a pregnancy when she wants one. In fact, many of the best diabetic clinics are now suggesting that this planning should even be taken to the point where sugar levels are controlled especially carefully in the months when trying to conceive. However, diabetes itself may complicate the choice of contraception.

One of the normally unimportant effects of the pill is that it slightly alters the way the body handles carbohydrates. This means that diabetic women (who already have difficulty in this) may find themselves needing slightly more insulin when starting the pill. Fortunately this does not seem to matter and does not affect the course of the diabetes. Some people have suggested that since both diabetes and the pill affect blood-vessels the pill should not be taken by diabetic women, but there is no proof of this.

However, some women prefer the IUCD. Recently there was a suggestion from Scotland that the IUCD failed more often in diabetic women. Nobody else has been able to prove this and, since some studies suggest the opposite, we see no reason to dissuade diabetic women from using the coil. Since diabetic women are said to be more prone to infectious disease than others the fact that the IUCD increases the risk of pelvic infections may be a more important consideration (see Chapter 7 for a fuller discussion of this).

Epileptics

Many couples in which one partner has epileptic fits are particularly worried about having children. Of course, epilepsy is not usually passed on to one's children and there is no reason why epileptic women should deprive themselves of a family for this reason. However, there is one snag to be aware of. Almost all the medicines which help prevent fits will also affect the use of the contraceptive pill. The reason for this is that the body gets used to breaking down medicines and breaks the pill down much too quickly. For

167

this reason a much higher dose of the pill is needed. This does not increase the risk of course because the amount of hormone going round the body remains the same. Most epileptic women find that they need a 50μg pill or even a 50 *and* a 30μg pill. Taking a relatively higher dose is no reason for them to be put off this method of contraception.

Alternative sources of family planning help

We have already implied in this book that while a woman's choice of contraception is up to her, it is useful for her to find a sympathetic adviser she can trust to help in making this decision. Sometimes this may be the doctor who looks after her general health problems but there may be times when she needs or wants to look elsewhere. We are going to finish this book with a few suggestions for finding alternative advisers. Some of these, such as family planning clinics, are open to everybody without a referral letter from their own family doctors. If, however, you wish to see a gynaecologist you may need to ask your general practitioner for a letter of referral. Sometimes if doctors are sure they are giving you the right advice they may be reluctant to refer you to a colleague. Do remember that you have the right to a second opinion. Ask for this tactfully but firmly.

General practitioners

Lots of people do not seem to realize that you can consult any General Practitioner who offers contraceptive ser- vices—it does not have to be the one who looks after the rest of your health care.

Community clinics

In Britain most health authorities run at least one family planning clinic that will be near to you. In the US the equivalents are the women's health clinics, or Planned Parenthood Clinics. Anyone can go to these clinics without being sent by their doctor. In the UK all treatment is free and the days are long since gone when the unmarried or under-16s were turned away. The doctors and nurses running these clinics are specialists in family planning and this can be especially useful if the decision is not straightforward. One difficulty is that since these clinics specialize in contraception they are often unable to deal with problems they pick up incidentally, such as thrush. Most will refer you back to your own doctor for treatment for these conditions. They may also be unnecessarily thorough in assessing you for contraception. There is no logical reason for an internal examination before starting on the pill but there are still some clinics that do this. Equally, other clinics are enthusiastic about performing cervical smears at unnecessarily frequent intervals. Perhaps the best suggestion we can make about this is to encourage the doctors to explain why they want to do a particular test or examination.

Brook advisory clinics

These family planning clinics operate mainly in the big cities of the United Kingdom. They were set up to help younger women, especially those under 20, and they are well known for their friendly, helpful approach. They are often willing to help with other crises in the life of the young, such as unwanted pregnancy and sexual difficulties. They are particularly recommended for the under-16s.

British Pregnancy Advisory Service (BPAS)

This organization was set up as a charity in Birmingham, but now has branches throughout Britain. It provides a fair and reasonable access to advice for women with unwanted pregnancies, and provides them with abortions where appropriate. Many of their branches now provide a contraceptive service and they also provide an easy to get to post-coital contraception service.

Pregnancy Advisory Service (PAS)

This London based organization also provides help for the woman with an unwanted pregnancy as well as morning-after contraception, which they have done a lot to publicize.

The Family Planning Association (FPA)

Although the FPA were the original founders of most of the Family Planning clinics in the United Kingdom, they handed them over to the National Health Service in 1974. They now run only a limited number of family planning clinics which are primarily for research. They do produce a lot of informative leaflets through FPIS (Family Planning Information Services) of 27–35 Mortimer Street, London W1.

The domiciliary family planning services

Most big cities in the UK now run family planning services that can take the doctors and nurses out to the home of the consumer. Few readers of this book will need them, but it is worth remembering them for those who are unable to leave the house because of family conditions or disease and for whom the general practitioner is unable to provide help.

Gynaecologists

A woman in the United States is more likely than her British counterpart to seek family-planning advice directly from her gynaecologist. Although some gynaecologists have a special interest in family planning, most of them are not really of much help in this area. Gynaecology is a big subject nowadays and many gynaecologists are busy concentrating on the surgical side of their speciality. The time they do come into their own is when there is a particular gynaecological problem complicating the method of contraception that someone has chosen. Usually it is best to accept the advice of a family doctor or clinic in going to see one. They are usually able to arrange the appointment.

Books

If we have whetted your appetite for more information about contraception you might like to try some of the following.

Guillebaud, John (1984), *The Pill*, 2nd edn, Oxford University Press.

Christopher, Elphis (1980), *Sexuality and birth control in social and community work*, Temple Smith, London.

Phillips, Angela and Rakusen, Jill (1978), *Our bodies ourselves*, Penguin, Harmondsworth.

Llewellyn-Jones, Derek (1980), *Everywoman*, Faber Paperbacks, London.

Index

Index

Index

Index

Index

Index